Genetic ByPass:

Using nutrition to bypass genetic mutations

By

Dr. Amy Yasko

Copyright © 2005 by Dr. Amy Yasko
Illustrations by Melissa Yasko

All rights reserved. This work, in whole or in part, may not be copied nor reproduced without express written permission of the authors.

Disclaimer: This information is presented by independent medical experts whose sources of information include studies from the world's medical and scientific literature, patient records, and other clinical and anecdotal reports. All dosages listed are based on the author's personal experiences. It is important to note that each person's body type and tolerance levels to supplements may be somewhat different. The publisher, author, and/or experts specifically cited in this publication are not responsible for any consequences, direct or indirect, resulting from any reader's action(s). This book is not intended to be a substitute for consultation with a health care provider. You, the reader, are instructed to consult with your personal health care provider prior to acting on any suggestions contained in this book. The purpose of this publication is to educate the reader. The material in this book is for informational purposes only and is not intended for the diagnosis or treatment of disease.

ISBN 0-9759674-3-6
Published by Matrix Development Publishing

Dedication

Occasionally an individual is fortunate enough to have a single supportive person in their lives. I am blessed to be surrounded by loving and supportive people in every aspect of my life. The support that I am given in both my work and home environments gives me the strength and the impetus to spend my time trying to help others to have optimal health and wellness.

In addition, the support I receive gives me the courage to bring forth new ideas. While it may not seem that this should require courage, believe me it does. Many in this universe operate from a position of fear. Fear of the unknown, fear of knowledge, and fear of new ideas. The goal of this book is to bring forth new ideas, to share knowledge and to help to remove the fear of genetic testing.

A thank you to Gloria and Dave for your unwavering love.

A special thank you to Garry and Alexandra for their love and for encouraging me to share my findings beyond the scope of my practice.

A very special thank you to Ed, Missie, Jessie and Cassie for giving me the strength, love, courage and confidence to help others to overcome their fears.

Contents

Part 1
General Background

Preface
The Basics
The Methylation Cycle for Nutrigenomic Analysis
The Importance of the Methylation Pathway
Overall Pathway Diagram
Descriptions of Specific Enzymes in the Pathway

Part 2

Nutritional Analysis for Specific SNPs
Additional Resources
Concluding Thoughts
About the Author
References

Part 1

General Background

Preface

Understanding Multifactorial Disease
Excerpt from Heal Your Body Naturally: The Power of RNA
By Dr. Amy Yasko and Dr. Garry Gordon

Once upon a time... life was a lot simpler. In today's society life is complex and so are our diseases. Years ago, in most families mom stayed at home and dad went to work. "The Donna Reed" show played on our black and white televisions. There were 40 million cars on the road in 1950, compared with over 225 million vehicles on the road as of the year 2000. That is close to a 600% increase in vehicles along with an equivalent increase in carbon monoxide, nitrogen dioxide, sulfur dioxide, benzene, formaldehyde, and polycyclic hydrocarbons from the exhaust of these vehicles.

Our environment has changed drastically since the 1950's. With the industrialization of the world, the amounts of toxic metals have increased markedly. In today's society, levels of lead, mercury and cadmium are all found to be in far greater concentrations than what is recommended for optimal health and longevity. These heavy metals are contributing to the epidemic of degenerative disease we are seeing today in every country in all age groups.

"Heavy metals are present in our air, drinking water, food, and countless human-made chemicals and products. They are taken into the body via inhalation, ingestions, and skin absorption. If heavy metals enter and accumulate in body tissues faster than the body's detoxification pathways can dispose of them, a gradual buildup of these toxins will occur. High-concentration exposure is not necessary to produce a state of toxicity in the body, as heavy metals accumulate in body tissues and, over time, can reach toxic concentration

levels. Human exposure to heavy metals has risen dramatically in the last 50 years as a result of an exponential increase in the use of heavy metals in industrial processes and products. Today, chronic exposure comes from mercury-amalgam dental fillings, lead-based paint, tap water, chemical residues in processed foods, and personal care products-cosmetics, shampoo and other hair products, mouthwash, toothpaste and soap. In today's industrial society, there is no escaping exposure to toxic chemicals and metals. In addition to the hazards both at home and outdoors, many occupations involve daily metal exposure. Over 50 professions entail exposure to mercury alone. These include physicians, pharmaceutical workers, any dental occupation, laboratory workers, hairdressers, painters, welders, metalworkers, battery makers, engravers, photographers, visual artists, and potters." (Pouls, M., Extreme Health, Univ. Michigan).

Toxic metals accumulate in our bodies over our lifetimes, beginning with the amounts we receive from our mothers during pregnancy; metals we are inoculated with during vaccination; and the metals we consume and breathe every day thereafter. Today, over 630,000 children are born each year with unsafe mercury levels, and that is even before we begin to vaccinate these children with injections containing mercury and aluminum. (EPA, Feb 5, 2004) It is clear to see that models of treatment that were based on a society that existed in the 1950's are outdated in terms of the needs of today's environmental milieu.

Fifty years ago we did not have the stress of two working parents in almost every household. The divorce rate has doubled since the 1950s, with more of us living in single parent households. Serving the role of both mom and dad creates additional stress. We have fast food, fast cars, and a fast pace of life with all the stressors that go with it. And all of that was before September 11, 2001. Now we have fears of terrorism in our own backyards to compound these other tensions in our lives.

The mid twentieth century saw the advent of antibiotics. While these medical treatments were successful for acute bacterial illness, those methods are not well suited for the prevalent chronic inflammatory conditions we encounter in the twenty first century. However, for the most part, our approach to disease has not changed drastically from that time.

"Medicine's molecular revolution is long overdue. By now, enthusiasts led us to believe, gene therapy and related treatments should have transformed clinical practice. Diseases, they told us, would be cured at their genetic roots, by repairing defective DNA or by disabling the genes of infectious microbes. But it has proved frustratingly difficult to make these methods work in the clinic, if you get sick, your doctor will probably still treat you with the pills and potions of old fashioned medicinal chemistry." (Check, E. Nature, Sept 2003.)

It has reached a point where it is not sufficient to merely take a drug for an illness. At one time it was enough to take an antibiotic to treat a bacterial infection. That is no longer the case. Antibiotic use has recently been associated with an increased risk of breast cancer. (Journal American Medical Assoc., February 18, 2004), and with an elevated risk of heart disease (Ray, W. New England J Medicine, Sept 9, 2004). No, the entire picture with respect to disease is not as straightforward as it once was.

The infectious disease landscape itself has also become more complex in spite of the advent of antibiotics and more the aggressive vaccination programs since the 1950's. We now talk in terms of the "total microbial or pathogen burden", and its effect upon an individual. It is not uncommon in this day and age for people to harbor a number of chronic bacterial and viral infections in their system simultaneously. These organisms can be seen as taking advantage of an unhealthy body to set up housekeeping in a system that has the right conditions to allow them to grow and flourish.

The issue is not the microbial organism per se, rather multisystem imbalances in the body that create an atmosphere that allows for the growth of these opportunistic organisms. This is not that dissimilar from termites infesting rotting wood. While this is a repulsive visual image, it makes the point that it is important to look at all aspects that effect health in your life, to prevent your body from becoming a veritable pillar of rotting wood that will allow the growth of the microbiological equivalent of termites in your system. A slightly less distasteful way to look at "opportunistic" organisms is to think of them in terms of their ability to take advantage of you. Opportunistic organisms are not unlike invaders in your home. Opportunistic organisms invade your body when it is vulnerable in the same way that an intruder will invade your home if it is unlocked with the front door left wide open! While it is still possible to have an intruder even with the best security precautions, you are less likely to have intruders if the front door is closed and locked. In a similar manner you may sometimes become ill even if you take excellent care of your body. However, we can reduce the risk of human invasion into our homes with proper prevention, just as we can reduce the risk of opportunistic microbial invasion in our bodies with proper attention to all aspects of our health.

In the book, "The Puzzle of Autism :Putting It All Together"(Gordon and Yasko, Matrix Development Publishing, 2004) the authors presented the hypothesis that chronic viral and bacterial organisms in our bodies are able to create additional havoc in your system by acting as "accomplices" to heavy metals, and aiding in their retention in the body. This adds yet another layer of complication to the story and again reiterates the fact that the diseases we face today are multifactorial and complex in nature.

We can attempt to lower the stress in our lives. However, for many of us the stress in our lives is a given, not a variable. While we may be able to affect <u>how</u> we react to the stress, we are unable to lower the total burden of stress that we are under. We can try to reduce our personal toxin burden, and our exposure to infectious diseases. Yet, unless we become like the "boy in the bubble" and isolate ourselves from our environment this becomes virtually impossible. We can eat organic foods, use only natural materials in our homes, use cleansers without chemicals, and eat chemical free foods, and drink filtered water. All of this adds another layer of complication and stress to our already overburdened lives. We still need to go out and interact in the world where everyone else <u>does not</u> create a chemical free, toxin free, microbe free environment. We can however do our best in each of these categories. If we can make even a small difference in every category of risk factors for disease, then we can reduce the likelihood of having disease.

Clearly, a number of factors contribute and interact to create the ultimate scenario of a diseased state. The more stressed your system and the greater your metal and toxic burden, the more likely you are to be harboring infectious organisms like bacteria, viruses and yeast. The number of infectious pathogens to which an individual has been exposed (infectious burden) has been correlated with a number of conditions, including coronary artery disease, gastric ulcers, and cervical cancer just to name a few. The proven and suspected roles of microbes is not limited to physical ailments; infections are increasingly being examined as associated causes of or possible contributors to a variety of serious, chronic neuropsychiatric disorders and to developmental problems, especially in children. (Institute of Medicine Report, Natl. Academies Press, June 2004).

"The problem with diabetes, hypertension, heart disease and other common ailments is untangling the genetic factors from a person's lifestyle and environment. What causes an individual's diabetes, overeating or bad genes? Human habits make it more challenging. Genetics certainly isn't the only factor in diseases. A hundred years ago, diabetes was much less of a problem, and in the last century human genes haven't changed much. What has changed, however, are eating habits and physical activity." (Berger, E. Houston Chronicle)

An extension of these concepts is that most disease we see today will in fact be multifactorial in nature. While we cannot change your genetic susceptibility, we can look at your genetic profile and use nutritional supplementation to help to bypass underlying genetic weaknesses to lower your genetic risk factors. This will help you to achieve optimal health when used in conjunction with a program to reduce some of the other risk factors such as environmental toxins and infectious agents.

The Basics

We have reached a point in today's society where every illness needs to be viewed from the standpoint of multifactorial disease. Many factors influence our susceptibility to disease. These include our stress load, our environment and the toxins we absorb from it, the total number of infectious agents we are exposed to as well as our underlying genetic susceptibility to these diseases. The precise combination of components that interact to cause multifactorial diseases may be different in every individual. There may be slight or enormous changes in the relative contributions of each of these components to disease. Multifactorial diseases are caused by infections and environmental events occurring in *genetically susceptible individuals*. Basic parameters like age and gender, along with other genetic and environmental factors, play a role in the onset of these diseases. Infections combined with excessive environmental burdens only lead to disease if they occur in individuals with the *appropriate genetic susceptibility*.

It is important in this day and age to address all of the contributing factors to these diseases. One clear, definitive way to evaluate the genetic contribution of multifactorial disease is to take advantage of new methodologies that allow for personalized genetic screening. Genetic testing gives us a way to evaluate and address the genetic component of multifactorial disease. Currently, tests are available to identify a number of underlying genetic susceptibilities based on allelic variations that are found in the DNA. Unfortunately, the use of this testing has fallen short of expectations. Perceived impediments to the use of genetic screening to identify underlying susceptibilities to disease include concerns of job discrimination, loss of insurance coverage and the inability to address diagnosed disease states.

While 79% of Americans surveyed responded that they would take a genetic test to assess the risks of inherited diseases, and 41% said they had a family history of genetic or inherited health problems, the reality is that genetic testing is severely under utilized. Genetic screening should be the wave of the future for both alternative healthcare as well as allopathic medicine. Both disciplines (alternative and allopathic medicine) should be taking advantage of the strides made in the Human Genome Project that allow us to utilize simple genetic tests to look at our genetic weaknesses.

The goal of the Human Genome Project was to identify all the approximately 30,000 genes in human DNA and to determine the sequences or "spelling" of the 3 billion chemical base pairs that make up human DNA. This project was completed in June of 2000. As a direct consequence of having the complete sequence of the human genome, research first focused on identifying particular genes that were involved with specific diseases. The next step has been to use this information to look for the presence of these identified disease causing genes in an individual person. Rather than looking at complete gene profiles, it is also possible to look at particular changes in the "spelling" of your DNA in only specific areas of interest. In this way, you can more quickly get a sense of known genetic weaknesses. In order to find relationships between genetic changes and the susceptibility to disease, this testing is done utilizing single nucleotide polymorphisms, otherwise known as SNPs (pronounced *snips*). This process systematically compares genomes of those individuals with a disease or an imbalance in a nutritional pathway to the corresponding DNA of a "normal" population.

If the potential of genetic testing is so great, and most Americans feel that they would be willing to take genetic tests, and that genetic issues affect their family's health, then why has this technology not been used to its full potential?

The answer is *FEAR*.

For most people a great fear exists that genetic screening will uncover a serious, fatal or life threatening condition. As a result individuals are fearful of the results of genetic screening. This points to the need to have a way to address the results of genetic screens so that we not only diagnose genetic susceptibility but also have a way to respond to it.

The lack of use of this powerful diagnostic technology highlights the need for adequate means to address the results of personalized genetic testing. It is a travesty to have the ability to specifically identify genetic weakness, yet have this technology underutilized out of fear. It points to a dire need for therapeutic technologies that take advantage of this same genetic information with an eye toward personalized treatment or nutritional supplementation, rather than simply personalized diagnosis. It is essential that we take advantage of the strides that have been made in the human genome project not only to understand our underlying genetic susceptibilities but also to successfully deal with chronic health issues.

The beauty of nutrigenomic testing is that it focuses on weaknesses in known, characterized nutritional pathways. Knowledge of these pathways lends itself to providing nutritional "bypasses" for genetic mutations.

These nutritional pathways can be viewed as complex roadways. Any mutations in the pathways can be visualized as road blocks. If we are familiar enough with the roadways and the maps we can design detours to get around the road blocks. The field of nutrigenomic testing and the supplementation of nutrients should take the fear out of genetic testing, at least for these well characterized nutritional pathways.

Nutrigenomics integrates concepts in molecular biology and genomics to study the ability of foods and nutritional supplements to interact with genes to influence our health and lower the genetic risk component for multifactorial disease. This field of nutrigenomics is perhaps best described by the group that is dedicated to promoting this new science of nutritional genomics. According to the National Center of Excellence in Nutritional Genomics at UC Davis, *"The science of nutrigenomics seeks to provide a molecular understanding for how common dietary chemicals (i.e., nutrition) affect health by altering the expression and/or structure of an individual's genetic makeup. Just as pharmacogenomics has led to the concept of "personalized medicine" and "designer drugs", so will the new field of nutrigenomics open the way for "personalized nutrition." In other words, by understanding our nutritional needs, our nutritional status, and our genotype, nutrigenomics should enable individuals to manage better their health and well-being by precisely matching their diets with their unique genetic makeup."*

The nutrigenomic test results that are analyzed in this book focus on genetic weaknesses in a particular pathway in the body that is involved in generating and utilizing methyl groups in the body. This central pathway in the body is particularly amenable to nutrigenomic screening for genetic weaknesses. Defects in methylation lay the appropriate groundwork for the further assault of environmental and infectious agents and result in an increased risk for additional health conditions including diabetes, cardiovascular disease, thyroid dysfunction, neurological inflammation, chronic viral infection, neurotransmitter imbalances, atherosclerosis, cancer, aging, neural tube defects, Alzheimer's disease and autism.

As a result of decreased activity in the methylation pathway due to mutations, there is a shortage of methyl groups in the body for a variety of important functions. Methyl groups are "CH3" groups that are moved around in the body to turn on or off genes. There are several particular sites in this pathway where blocks can occur as a result of genetic weaknesses. Supplementation with appropriate foods and nutrients will bypass these mutations to allow for restored function of the pathway.

By looking at diagrammatic representations of the methylation pathway and relating the effects of genetic polymorphisms to biochemical pathways, we are able to draw a personalized map for each individual's imbalances which may impact upon their health. By identifying the precise areas of genetic fragility, it is then possible to target appropriate nutritional supplementation of these pathways to optimize the functioning of these crucial biochemical processes.

"With the completion of the Human Genome Project, we have a nearly complete list of the genes needed to produce a human. However the situation is far more complex than a simple catalogue of genes. Of equal importance is a second system that cells use to determine when and where a particular gene will be expressed during development. This system (DNA methylation) *is overlaid on DNA in the form of epigenetic marks that are heritable during cell division but do not alter the DNA....The importance of DNA methylation is emphasized by the growing number of human diseases that are known to occur when this epigenetic information is not properly established and /or maintained..."*

Keith Robertson, Nature Review Genetics, August 2005.

The Methylation Cycle for Nutrigenomic Analysis

The methylation cycle is the ideal pathway to focus on for nutrigenomic analysis and supplementation because the function of this pathway is essential for a number of critical reactions in the body. As a consequence, genetic weaknesses (mutations) in this pathway are risk factors for a number of serious health conditions including heart disease, stroke, cancer, diabetes, MS, Alzheimer's disease, ALS, Parkinson's disease, Huntington's disease, CFS/FM, mitochondrial disease, SLE, neural tube defects, miscarriages, Down's syndrome, bipolar disorder, schizophrenia, repair of tissue damage, proper immune function, the aging process as well as autism. In the field of autism, which is my major area of study at this time, I have genetic data on almost 200 individuals. Thus far 100% of the children show one or more mutations somewhere in this pathway. Even if this percentage does not hold up over time, I would expect that a statistically significant number of children with autism will harbor mutations in this pathway.

Methylation is related to neurotransmitter levels; methylation of intermediates in tryptophan metabolism can affect the levels of serotonin; intermediates of the methylation pathway are also shared with the pathway involved in serotonin and dopamine synthesis. Consequently, imbalances in the methylation pathway will also affect the neurotransmitter dopamine. In addition to its direct role as a neurotransmitter, dopamine is involved in methylating phospholipids in the cell membranes to increase membrane fluidity. Membrane fluidity is important for a variety of reasons including proper signaling of the immune system as well as protecting nerves from damage. A number of serious neurological conditions site reduced membrane fluidity as part of the disease process including MS, ALS, and Alzheimer's disease. In addition, phospholipid methylation may be involved in modulation of NMDA (glutamate) receptors, acting to control excitotoxin damage.

Increases in certain inflammatory mediators of the immune system such as IL6 and TNF alpha lead to decreases in methylation. Chronic inflammation would therefore exacerbate an existing genetic condition of undermethylation. The inability to progress normally through the methylation pathway as a result of this methylation cycle mutation, could lead to a build up of precursors of the methylation pathway, including the excitotoxin glutamate.

The building blocks for DNA and RNA require the methylation pathway. Without adequate DNA and RNA it is difficult for the body to synthesize new cells. This would result in a decreased level of new cells including critical cells of the immune system, the T cells. De novo T cell synthesis is necessary to respond to bacterial, parasitic and viral infection, as well as for other aspects of the proper functioning of the immune system. T cells are necessary for antibody producing cells in the body (B cells) as both T helpers and T suppressors are needed to appropriately regulate the antibody response.

In addition, decreased levels of methylation can result in improper DNA regulation. DNA methylation is necessary to prevent the expression of viral genes that have been inserted into the body's DNA. Loss of methylation can lead to the expression of inserted viral genes.

Proper levels of methylation are also directly related to the body's ability to both myelinate nerves and to prune nerves. Myelin is a sheath that wraps around the neuronal wiring to insulate and facilitate faster transmission of electrical potentials. Without adequate methylation, the nerves cannot myelinate in the first place, or cannot remyelinate after insults such as viral infection or heavy metal toxicity. A secondary effect of a lack of methylation and hence decreased myelination is inadequate pruning of nerves. Pruning helps to prevent excessive wiring of unused neural connections and reduces the synaptic density. Without adequate pruning the brain cell connections are misdirected and proliferate into dense, bunched thickets. All of these changes, when they occur in utero or in very young children, can alter brain development and can also set up metabolic changes that cause ongoing compromise of brain function. These metabolically caused changes in brain function can, however, be mitigated if the underlying nutrigenomic weaknesses that are causing these changes are identified and supplemented nutritionally.

We are used to talking about single biomarkers serving as indicators for specific disease states. However, I believe that for a number of health conditions, including autism, we may be looking at the entire methylation pathway (as it is drawn on the diagrams presented in this book) as representing "the biomarker" for underlying genetic susceptibility for a number of disease states. We may then need to expand our view of a "biomarker" beyond the restriction of a mutation in a single gene to a mutation somewhere in an entire pathway of interconnected function.

This does not mean that every individual with mutations in this pathway will be autistic or will have one of the health conditions listed above. It may be a necessary but not a sufficient condition. As described in the Preface and The Basics section of this book, most health conditions that we see today are multifactorial in nature. There are genetic components, infectious components and environmental components. A certain threshold or body burden needs to be met for each of these factors in order for multifactorial disease to occur. However part of what makes the methylation cycle so unique and so critical for our health, is that mutations in this pathway have the capability to impair all three of these factors. This would suggest that if an individual has enough mutations or weaknesses in this pathway it MAY be sufficient to cause mutlifactorial disease, as methylation cycle mutations can lead to chronic infectious diseases, increased environmental toxin burdens and have secondary effects on genetic expression.

Brief overview of potential consequences of variations in the genes in the methylation pathway including:

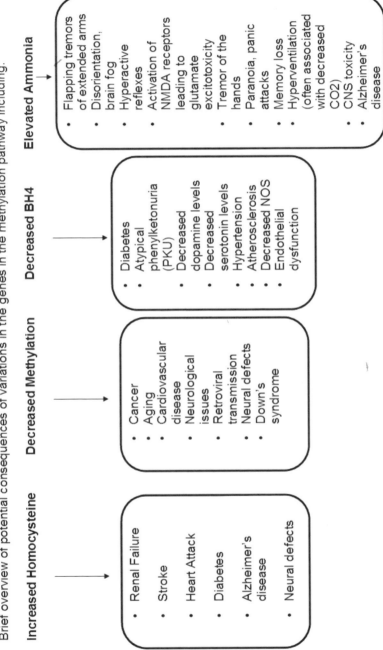

Increased Homocysteine
- Renal Failure
- Stroke
- Heart Attack
- Diabetes
- Alzheimer's disease
- Neural defects

Decreased Methylation
- Cancer
- Aging
- Cardiovascular disease
- Neurological issues
- Retroviral transmission
- Neural defects
- Down's syndrome

Decreased BH4
- Diabetes
- Atypical phenylketonuria (PKU)
- Decreased dopamine levels
- Decreased serotonin levels
- Hypertension
- Atherosclerosis
- Decreased NOS
- Endothelial dysfunction

Elevated Ammonia
- Flapping tremors of extended arms
- Disorientation, brain fog
- Hyperactive reflexes
- Activation of NMDA receptors leading to glutamate excitotoxicity
- Tremor of the hands
- Paranoia, panic attacks
- Memory loss
- Hyperventilation (often associated with decreased CO_2)
- CNS toxicity
- Alzheimer's disease

The Importance of the Methylation Pathway

- **Methylation and Nucleic Acid Synthesis**

  New cell synthesis and repair

  Mutations in the methylation pathway can cripple the ability of the body to make the building blocks (purines and pyrimidines) needed for new DNA and RNA synthesis. A reduced capacity for new DNA and RNA synthesis means that any new cell synthesis is impaired. For an organism to live, it must create new cells as fast as cells die. This requires that the body make millions of cells every minute, relying on DNA and RNA synthesis.

  A reduced synthesis capacity due to methylation cycle mutations is a particular issue for cells that already have difficulties meeting their needs for DNA and RNA synthesis under normal conditions. For instance, bone marrow cells, lymphocytes, erythrocytes and some brain cells cannot make some of the DNA and RNA bases that they need for synthesis. Intestinal mucosa cells cannot make enough purines to fulfill the body's requirement. Stress increases the need for nucleotides to overcome negative effects of hormones released during stressful conditions. Cell repair after injury increases the need for nucleotides. The brain has the highest concentration of RNA in the body, and therefore has the highest requirement of RNA.

  Problems in the methylation pathway limit nucleotide building blocks that the brain and other organs need for repair and growth.

RNA based regulation

Universal lack of methylation and the inability to produce nucleic acids necessary for RNA synthesis results in a situation where the body is lacking the required regulatory elements for RNA based genetic silencing. Silencing is a multistep process that involves RNA as well as methylation and deacetylation of histones.

In addition there is a direct tie between RNAi (RNA interference) and DNA methylation; double stranded RNA can induce DNA methylation.

- **DNA Methylation**

CpG Methylation

Epigenetic modification of DNA occurs mainly on cytosine nucleotides. Cytosine is one of the four DNA bases found in organisms, including humans. Methylation of cytosine is generally correlated with silencing of genes. In humans, this methyl group is found on the 5 position of cytosines that precede guanosine in CpG dinucleotides. One difference between bacterial and human genomes is that bacterial genes are *not* methylated at specific CpG regions. Research has shown that when mammalian genes are not methylated at CpG regions it can trick the immune system into reacting against itself and causing autoimmunity.

It has been estimated that 70 to 80% of the CpG sites are methylated in humans. The other 20% of the CpGs that are not methylated are found in clusters known as "islands". These nonmethylated CpG islands are most often found in the region that turns on the gene, known as the promoter region. Thus methylation of C's creates two distinct regions in the

DNA, "unmethylated CpG islands" and "methylated CpG sites" that are distributed throughout the genome. These CpG methylated regions tend to be located at mutational hot spots; one third of all point mutations (single base changes) associated with cancer are at these sites.

Once these cytosine nucleotides are methylated they are able to undergo a reaction to form the base thymidine which creates a single base change in the DNA sequence. It is not known if underlying mutations in the overall methylation pathway which lead to decreased levels of thymidine have any influence on the rate at which this reaction occurs.

Methylation of cytosine also helps to maintain the large amount of noncoding human DNA in an inert state as well as helping to silence harmful DNAs. If you are short on methyl groups due to methylation cycle mutations then you will have less methyl groups for preventing autoimmunity and silencing genomes. This is true for silencing viral genomes as well as for regulating your own DNA.

Methylation of Viral DNA

DNA methylation helps to maintain the large amount of non-coding DNA in an inert state. This is applicable to the DNA or genome of the organism, as well as any viral genes that are harbored within the cell. The methylation process prevents the transcription (the reading) of inserted viral sequences. One of the consequences of loss of methylation function is that it could cause the potentially harmful expression of these inserted viral genes. Under-methylation in normally silent regions of the DNA can cause the expression of inserted viral genes.

Methylation of Host Organism DNA

Methylation is important for turning on and off mammalian DNA. This is true for silencing viral DNA in the body as well as cellular DNA. There are sections of the DNA prior to the information or coding portion that contain regulatory sequences or sections. When these regulatory regions are methylated properly they turn on and off the information portions as they should. During development DNA methylation patterns are established and are essential for normal development. During new cell synthesis these patterns are then replicated. When these regions do not have the correct amount of methyl groups bound to them it can prevent the information from being turned off, resulting in autoimmunity, aging and cancer.

Methylation and Trinucleotide Repeat Disorders

Certain disease states occur as a result of increases in the length of specific three base repeat sections in the genome. These special "repeat regions" are prior to the information or coding region of the DNA. These trinucleotide repeats are involved in certain disorders such as Friedreich's ataxia, Fragile X and Huntington's disease. We also see a role for trinucleotide repeats in particular regions of genes that serve regulatory purposes, such as the reelin gene that is involved in myelination.

When there is insufficient methylation capacity (mutations in the pathway) there is often not enough methyl groups to bind to these repeat regions, so they are able to multiply. This results in very long repeat sections, much longer than they should be. Studies have shown that inhibition of DNA methylation resulted in a 1000 fold increase in these three base repeat sections. Therefore, decreased DNA methylation results in increases in trinucleotide repeats and increases the risks for these disorders.

These long repeated sections then attract the limited methyl groups that are available. The consequent overmethylation of these repeat sections results in shutting off genes inappropriately.

Methylation and the X Chromosome

Females contain two copies of the X chromosome. Silencing one of these two copies is essential for normal development. Methylation of the DNA is the mechanism by which the second X chromosome is silenced. The normally nonmethylated "CpG islands" become methylated as part of this silencing process.

A similar strategy is utilized to silence one of two copies of genes other than those on the X chromosome. In these cases the inactivated (or imprinted) gene that is inactivated by methylation can be of either maternal or paternal origin. Loss of normal imprinting as a result of decreased methylation contributes to a number of inherited diseases including Beckwith-Wiedemann, Prader-Willi and Angelman syndromes, among others.

Methylation of Histone DNA

The expression of many cellular genes is modulated by histone acetylation in addition to DNA methylation. Interestingly, methylation also plays a role in the histone acetylation process. Methylation causes a hypoacetylation of histones H3 and H4 within the transgene suggesting that methylated DNA represses local transcription by recruiting histone deacetylase activity. Methylation also plays a pivotal role in establishing and maintaining an inactive state of a gene by rendering the chromatin structure inaccessible to the transcription machinery. Methylation therefore plays an important role in development, imprinting, X-chromosome inactivation and tissue-specific gene expression. Changes in DNA methylation profiles are common features of development and in a number of human diseases.

- **Methylation, Pregnancy and Neural Tube Defects**

Preconceptional supplementation to support the methylation cycle helps to prevent miscarriages. Mutations in the MTHFR genes of the methylation pathway as well as mutations that lead to decreased B12 are risk factors for neural tube defects. Mutations in the methylation pathway, specifically methionine synthase, methionine synthase reductase as well as elevated homocysteine are risk factors for having a child with Down's syndrome.

It is important to consider methylation pathway mutations when looking at supplementing folate during pregnancy. One way to understand this more easily is to think about the studies on folate and neural tube defects. Using folate during pregnancy helps to decrease the risk of neural tube defects. This is not changing the DNA but having a regulatory effect on the ability of the DNA to be expressed, known as epigenetics. Now, if folate can make a difference in DNA expression, but you have a mutation so that you cannot use folate, then taking folate may not do any good; it is almost as if you never supplemented at all. Running a nutrigenomic test to determine the form of folate that will bypass mutations in your folate pathway will enable you to supplement with the appropriate form of folate and should help to reduce the risk of neural tube defects in a similar way to the use of plain folate in the absence of mutations in this pathway.

The genetics of the parent are reflected in the child. So that if a pregnant mother has mutations that make her unable to utilize plain folate, you should consider testing the infant for similar weaknesses in this pathway. The sooner that you know if and where a newborn's genetic weaknesses reside in the methylation pathway the sooner you can start to supplement to bypass these mutations. Remember by supplementing properly you should have the potential to bypass and compensate for the mutations. If this is commenced from day one you do not allow time for virus to build up (remember that methylation is necessary to silence virus). In addition, some of the mutations in the methylation cycle make it difficult to make new T cells which are a critical part of your immune system. If chronic virus is not building then it cannot hang onto and store heavy metals. This should help to prevent huge stores of metals in the chronic virus in the system. If as suspected, virus and metal loads from vaccines are related to the autism epidemic and if a newborn does have some weakness in their methylation pathway, you have the option of supplementing with the appropriate nutrients prior to vaccination. This may make it easier for the immune system of infants to react to vaccines in the correct fashion.

If the methylation cycle is working properly from day one it should help with myelination, immune regulation, the ability to make new DNA and RNA that is needed for growing cells.

- **Methylation and Heart Disease**

Adequate levels of CoQ10 have been identified as necessary nutrients to help prevent congestive heart failure. Clinically CoQ10 has been used in the treatment of angina, heart failure prevention of reperfusion injury after coronary artery bypass and cardiomyopathy. The synthesis of CoQ10 in the body requires components of the methylation pathway; in particular it requires adequate levels of SAMe that is generated by the methylation cycle. Cholesterol lowering drugs (statin drugs) decrease the level of CoQ10 in the body. It may be particularly important for individuals taking statin drugs to be aware of the methylation status in their body and replenish CoQ10.

In addition, the relationship between elevated homocysteine levels, an increased risk of heart disease and the genetic risk associated with MTHFR C677T mutations in the methylation pathway has been recognized for quite some time. Appropriate supplementation of the methylation pathway should be able to help compensate for this mutation.

- **Methylation and Energy Production**

The mitochondria are the energy producing organelles within each cell. Decreased mitochondrial energy has been implicated in chronic fatigue, fibromyalgia and mitochondrial disease. Coenzyme Q10 is also important for its role in ATP production in the mitochondrial respiratory chain. Again, as mentioned above, methylation pathway function is necessary for the synthesis of CoQ10 in the body.

Carnitine is another nutrient produced by the body that is involved in mitochondrial energy production. Mitochondria fatty acid oxidation is the main energy source for heart and skeletal muscle. Carnitine is also involved in the transport of these fatty acids into the mitochondrial matrix. As with CoQ10, the synthesis of carnitine by the body requires methylation pathway function. Synthesis of carnitine begins with the methylation of the amino acid L-lysine by SAM, so once again we have a connection to the methionine/homocysteine pathways.

Another connection between carnitine and the methylation cycle is that an enzyme that is needed for carnitine synthesis is also utilized as part of a secondary route to form methionine from homocysteine. When there are methylation cycle mutations that impair the primary route of synthesis for methionine, this secondary route will be used more heavily. This can divert the enzyme from its ability to synthesize carnitine. Two recent studies suggest that this enzyme has a preference for the methylation pathway reaction (choline-TMG conversion), and that choline supplementation may decrease carnitine synthesis. Therefore it may be of greater benefit to supplement the methylation pathway with TMG rather than its precursor, choline.

Low muscle tone and extreme muscle weakness may in part be due to decreased mitochondrial energy as well as myelination problems due to reduced methylation cycle capacity.

Methylation is also needed to convert guanido acetic acid (guanido Ac) to methyl guanido acetate or creatine in the body. The methyl group for this reaction is donated by SAMe. As a next step within the muscle, creatine is then converted to creatine phosphate which acts as an energy reservoir helping to donate its phosphate group for the conversion of ADP to ATP under anaerobic conditions. In addition to its role in muscle energy, creatine has also been reported to play a role in speech, language, attention span and ability to follow commands. The conversion of guanido Ac to creatine is part of the same pathway that goes on to form creatinine. Changes in creatinine levels appear to reflect the ability to address chronic viral infection in the body.

- **Methylation and ADD**

    Some literature suggests that ADD/ADHD can be helped by the addition of SAMe. SAMe is a critical intermediate in the methylation cycle. SAMe is also a methyl donor for reactions that involve dopamine, epinephrine and norepinephrine. Imbalances in this biochemical region, dopamine, epinephrine and norepinephrine have been implicated in ADD/ADHD. One can envision that methylation cycle function is needed to produce SAMe as a methyl donor for the dopamine / norepinephrine / epinephrine pathways to help to prevent ADD/ADHD.

    COMT is another central enzyme that is involved in the methylation pathway. The high activity form of this enzyme that breaks down dopamine (COMT) has been associated with ADHD.

- **Protein Methylation**

    Protein methylation is reported to be analogous to protein phosphorylation. Both of these regulatory mechanisms appear to serve as molecular switches controlling protein activity and location in a reversible manner.

- **Methylation and Myelin**

    Myelin coating on nerve is important for proper neurotransmission. Methylation of amino acids in myelin basic protein helps to stabilize it against degradation. In animal studies the developmental increase in methylation capacity is correlated with parameters of myelination. Decreased levels of methylation acitivty in these animal models are related to conditions of demyelination.

• Methylation and the Immune System

New T cell synthesis is needed in order for T cell clones to expand and respond properly to an immune assault. T cells are needed to help to control the B cells and to balance TH1 and TH2 responses. If there are methylation cycle problems or mutations, you may have trouble making the bases that are needed for new DNA synthesis. If you cannot make new DNA, then you cannot make new T cells and as a result you may lack immune system regulatory cells.

The immune system has the B cell "arm" that makes antibodies, known as humoral immunity and the T cell "arm" known as cellular immunity. If you are having trouble making new T cells, then the immune response may become more heavily weighted in the direction of B cells. The B cells have the ability to respond by making antibody, or auto antibody rather than making the range of T cells that regulate as well as fight infections. B cell clones expand and then are available for the future. So there is a somewhat greater need for new DNA synthesis for the T cell response than for the B cell response.

In addition, individuals with methylation cycle mutations are more at risk as they will have problems making regulatory T cells that help the body to control the B cells and prevent autoimmune antibodies. Auto antibodies can occur as a result of imbalances in immune regulation. If you are not making adequate T cells (methylation pathway mutations) then you may lack regulatory T cells and can end up with auto antibodies.

Methylation also plays a role in the ability of the immune system to recognize foreign bodies or antigens that it needs to respond to. Research has shown that methylation is decreased in humans with auto immune conditions. Impaired methylation of T cells may be involved in the production of auto antibodies. Studies from patients with systemic lupus erythrematosis (SLE) have shown that their T cells are undermethylated. Impaired methylation of T cells may also be involved in the production of auto antibodies.

As proper methylation function is restored, it should help in regaining immune function regulation. In several cases I have seen the level of auto antibodies decline after proper methylation cycle supplementation.

Methylation of DNA is also used to regulate immune cells. Immune receptor DNA is initially in the "OFF" state and is maintained that way until the immune cells need to differentiate. At that time the methyl groups are removed from the DNA in a highly regulated fashion.

- **Methylation and Cancer**

Undermethylation of the entire genome is referred to as global hypomethylation. Global hypomethylation when it is paired with over methylation of highly select repeated regions of the gene is associated with both aging and cancer.

Both undermethylation of tumor causing genes (no turn OFF) and overmethylaiton of tumor suppressing genes (turned OFF) have been well characterized as contributing factors to cancer.

Methylation is used to inactivate excess levels of endogenous products that may be harmful to the body. For instance, excess estrogen is inactivated by methylation, with SAMe donating a methyl group for this process. The inability to inactivate excess estrogen has been linked to an increased susceptibility to hormone sensitive cancers.

Epidemiologic and mechanistic evidence suggests mutations in the methylation pathway are involved in colorectal neoplasia. Specifically the role of the MTHFR C677T and MTHFR A1298C, methionine synthase (MTR A2756G), methionine synthase reductase (MTRR A66G), cystathionine beta synthase (CBS exon 8, 68-base-pair insertion), and thymidylate synthase (TS enhancer region and 3'untranslated region) have been implicated in colorectal cancer.

- **Methylation and Allergic Reactions**

When methylation is impaired it can lead to abnormally high levels of histamine. High levels of histamine are causative factors in allergic reactions. Optimal methylation function is needed to break down histamine so that it does not build up in the body.

In addition to the effect of methylation on histamine levels, the effect of methyl groups on the TH1/TH2 balance may be a second mechanism by which decreased methylation may increase allergies. There are two sets of T helper cells in the immune system, TH1 and TH2 cells. While TH1 cells are involved in cell mediated immune responses and toning down or regulating TH2 activity, the TH2 cells have been associated with humoral or B cell mediated responses and allergic responses. TH2 cells trigger the activation and recruitment of IgE antibody producing B cells, mast cells and eosinophils that are involved in allergic inflammation. Studies show that decreased methylation of CpG regions in these genes may influence the balance of TH1 and TH2 cells.

- **Methylation and Anesthesia**

The level of various metabolites of the methylation pathway are important for protection from side effects of anesthesia. As early as 1942 it was recognized that the addition of methionine is preventative for side effects from the use of chloroform. Methionine affords protection from liver injury as a result of chloroform anesthesia. Methionine also protects against effects of nitrous oxide anesthesia. Nitrous oxide disrupts the activity of methionine synthase, a central enzyme in the methylation cycle. Again, preloading with methionine appears to accelerate recovery and reduce side effects associated with this form of anesthesia. The neurological deterioration and death of an infant boy has been reported who had been anesthetized twice within a short time with the anesthetic nitrous oxide. Postmortem studies determined that this child had a deficiency of the MTHFR which is a principle enzyme in the methylation pathway.

- **Methylation and Environmental Toxins**

Methylation is also required to clear environmental toxins from the body. This process involves conjugating methyl groups to the toxins prior to removal. Most of the methyl groups that are used for detoxification are donated by S adenosyl methionine (SAMe).

Nutritional support for the methylation pathway was able to prevent strychnine induced seizures and death in animal models, as well as to be protective against carbon tetrachloride induced toxicity. Supplementation was also able to prevent ethanol induced decreases in methylation cycle function.

Elimination of inorganic arsenic from the body requires methylation. After methylation arsenic can be eliminated from the body in the urine.

Differences in methylation may also account for susceptibility of different tissues to cadmium toxicity. In animal studies, methylation was necessary to induce metallothionein activity that was required for cadmium excretion.

The methylation process is also the major means of detoxifying selenium in the body.

Compounding the situation, environmental toxins are also able to have an negative impact on methylation. In experimental models, exposure of animals to environmental toxins during development appears to alter the pattern of DNA methylation. This change in DNA methylation is then maintained into future generations of offspring. The heavy metals, arsenic, nickel and chromium are able to cause over methylation of DNA. This can result in turning "OFF" of important regulatory genes such as tumor suppressor genes. In addition other environmental contaminants such as polycyclic aromatic hydrocarbons (PAH) and benzo(a)pyrene diol epoxide (BPDE) are able to bind to methylated CpG regions of the DNA. Cadmium also inhibits the methylation of phospholipids, interfering with cellular membrane functions.

- **Methylation and Aging**

    Intermediates of the methylation pathway are known to decrease with age along with a decline in methylation pathway function. DNA methylation is also known to decrease with aging. Age related decreases in methylation can lead to decreased methylation of T cells which may in part explain changes in immune function with age. Age related decreases in methylation can result in increased levels of homocysteine, increasing the risk of arthritis, cancer depression and heart disease. This would suggest that increasing the body's level of methylation through supplementation may extend healthy life span.

- **Methylation Affects Both Nature and Nurture**

    The overwhelming impact of methylation pathway mutations is exemplified by the July 9, 2005 article in Science News which reported that although identical twins have the identical DNA they often have differences in a number of traits including disease susceptibility. This study suggests that as twins go through life the environmental influences to which they are exposed affects which genes are actually turned on or off. Methyl or acetyl groups can attach to the DNA in a similar way that charms attach to a charm bracelet. This modification of the DNA is known as epigenetic regulation. The combination of environmentally determined addition of these "charms" to the bracelet of DNA, combined with inherited DNA changes or mutations lead to an individuals susceptibility to disease. According to the scientist who headed this study, Dr. Manuel Estseller, "My belief is that people are 50 percent genetics and 50 percent environment."

This statement should give us some understanding as to why mutations in the methylation pathway can be so devastating. Mutations in the methylation pathway affect the 50% of the pure genetic susceptibility; this would be analogous to defects in the links of the chain of our charm bracelet. In addition, because methylation is also necessary for the epigenetic modification of the DNA, methylation also affects the environmental 50%. If we take the analogy a step further to really understand the global impact of defects in this pathway we can view genetically inherited mutations in the methylation pathway as causing problems in the links of the bracelet and environmental effects creating a problem with the ability to put charms on the bracelet of DNA. Problems in the methylation pathway therefore can affect 100% of our susceptibility to disease. This is why it is critical for health to understand where our weaknesses in this pathway reside and then supplement appropriately to bypass these mutations.

DNA Bracelet

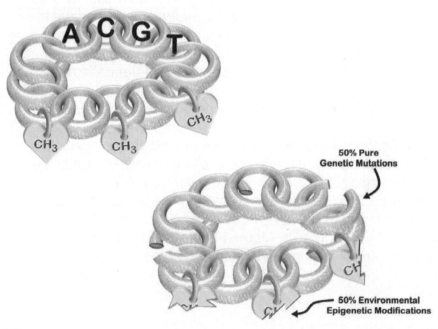

A second study that has also addressed the nature versus nurture question used animal models to look at this issue. Researchers were able to show that the adult response to stressful situations was heavily influenced by the interactions these same animals had as pups with their mothers at birth. Those pups with higher levels of care showed differences in the methylation patterns of stress related genes when compared with pups in the lower care test group. Dr. Szyf from the team at McGill University that conducted the study has stated that their study results "...have bridged the gap, nurture is nature."

This work does suggest that the bridge between "nature and nurture" is the ability of nurturing to influence DNA methylation. However, nurture alone cannot be the answer. According to this study nurturing can influence epigenetic modification of DNA, so nurturing can affect the number of "charms on the bracelet". However if there are genetic mutations in the DNA sequence itself, the actual "links of the bracelet" this will also affect the overall methylation capacity in the body. Without the mechanisms to produce the methyl groups, all of the nurturing in the world will not be able to overcome the lack in the production capacity for methylation. In other words if the body cannot produce the charms for the bracelet it becomes a moot point how easily you are able to attach them to the bracelet. Nutrigenomic support to bypass these mutations is necessary to address the weaknesses in the DNA that would result in reduced capacity in this pathway.

The Overall Methylation Pathway

What I am calling the "Methylation Pathway" in this book refers to the diagram on the following page. This diagram depicts the intersection between the methionine, the folate, the tetrahydrobiopterin (BH4), the urea and the Kreb's cycles in the body and interrelationships between these cycles as I see them. I think that part of the key to recognizing the importance of this pathway is the way in which you put the cycles together, and then recognizing that any mutation that impairs the function of these cycles is a risk factor for health issues. It may be that until now, no one has linked these cycles together in this way, so they have not recognized that *any* mutation in these cycles, as I have drawn them, is a risk factor for certain conditions including autism. This unique coupling of pathways has made it possible to recognize that mutations *anywhere* in this pathway can compromise critical functions in the body. It is common to think of biomarkers as a defect in a single gene causing a health condition. I think that in this case it is not a *single* mutation, rather a mutation *somewhere* in this pathway that impairs its function. While it is common to see the methionine and folate cycles linked, I find that by including BH4 recycling and the urea cycle it enables one to look at the overall impact and ramifications of a number of mutations in this pathway in a manner that may have previously been underappreciated. We are then able to see this entire interconnected "methylation" pathway as I have drawn it as the biomarker for a number of health conditions. I am asking you to think beyond the narrow concept of a single gene as representing a single biomarker for susceptibility. By arranging these cycles such that they interact as shown, we are able to understand the domino effects of specific mutations in these pathways. It then allows for the larger more global view that defects anywhere in this pathway serve as the underlying risk factors or biomarkers for health.

40

This methylation pathway diagram is a work in progress designed to help you to visualize how the folate, methionine, BH4 cycle, urea cycle and even the Krebs cycle are interconnected and how they relate to the various nutrigenomic mutations that can be screened for in this pathway. It should also help you to see where you can supplement these pathways, where the enzymes are located and where the mutations occur that impair the proper functioning of these pathways. In addition I have noted some of the steps in these pathways that are affected by toxic metals. You should be able to see how mutations and metals can work together to create a synergistic problem.

Based on the wide range of mutations that can occur in this pathway and the "domino effect" of mutations on the remainder of the pathway I feel that it is a wise idea to supplement small amounts of nutrients at a number of points in this pathway to ensure that the pathway will function to the best of its ability.

There are some basic types of supplementation that should be beneficial for anyone. I suggest supporting with 5 methyl THF to support the forward reaction of the MTHFR enzyme as well as to support mutations in the reverse reaction of this enzyme that impact levels of BH4 in the body.

The use of 5 formyl THF will feed directly into the points of the pathway that synthesize the DNA and RNA bases, known as nucleotides. As already discussed, nucleotides, DNA and RNA are critical for new cell synthesis and cellular repair. Due to the essential role that these nucleic acids and their building blocks serve in the body it is wise to supplement these compounds in a redundant fashion. In addition to the use of 5 formyl THF, I suggest that you directly add nucleotides to take some strain off of the pathway. Supplementation with specific RNAs will also be beneficial in terms of adding more complete

RNA molecules so that the pathway does not need work to produce RNA sequences under conditions where the body is lacking components of the required synthetic pathway for these essential molecules.

The addition of low doses of TMG (trimethyl glycine) and phosphatidyl serine or phosphatidyl choline help to support the secondary pathway going from homocysteine directly to methionine, bypassing the function of methionine synthase (MTR) and methionine synthase reductase (MTRR); the addition of B12, using the specific type dictated by genetics also helps to take some of the strain off of MTR and MTRR. On a related note, I have found by experience that B12 levels are related to potty training. Once you have supported the methylation pathway properly and are supplementing B12 to the level dictated by the mutations potty training and bowel control emerges. B12 is also helpful in balancing the body to address peripheral neuropathy as well as certain types of OCD behaviors.

Small amounts of plain methionine and, if indicated by genetics, the addition of SAMe (s adenosyl methionine) help to support at additional steps of these cycles. SAMe is often referred to as the universal methyl donor, as it provides the methyl groups for DNA, RNA, histones, neurotransmitters, membrane phospholipids, proteins, melatonin and numerous small molecules.

The goal is to use low doses of a variety of supplements to support a number of points of the pathway. I have found that this is easier on the system than using high doses of just a few supplements for this pathway. One way to understand this concept is to think of mutations in the pathway as accidents on a roadway. While it is possible to use a bulldozer to clear an accident that approach causes a great deal of collateral damage. On the other hand, if you recognize that there is more than one way to get from point A to point B, that you can take the highway, a second major roadway, a side road and a number of back roads, this opens up more gentle approaches to addressing the "accident" on the freeway. If you look to clear or bypass the accident as well as ensuring that all of the alternate routes are supported properly then you are more likely to keep traffic flowing in spite of the blockade on your major highway. The philosophy here is to recognize the pathways involved, the way in which they are interconnected and then supplement with small amounts of a number of nutrients to support the overall health of the entire pathway.

    It is important to keep in mind as you begin to supplement or bypass your genetic weaknesses in this pathway, that this pathway is also involved in the ability to silence viral infections and to detoxify environmental toxins and heavy metals. As you support this pathway, so that it functions properly, perhaps for the first time in your life, it may help your body to trigger natural detoxification mechanisms. While detoxification is important for overall long term health and wellness there can be temporary discomforts associated with the detoxification process. This is another reason to use the more gentle approach of supplementing with low doses of a number of supplements, rather than using the bulldozer approach. There are simple noninvasive tests that can be utilized to monitor the rate of excretion of toxins from your system as you support your body to bypass methylation cycle mutations. As you detoxify you begin to lower the environmental contributions to risk factors that affect your long term health and wellness.

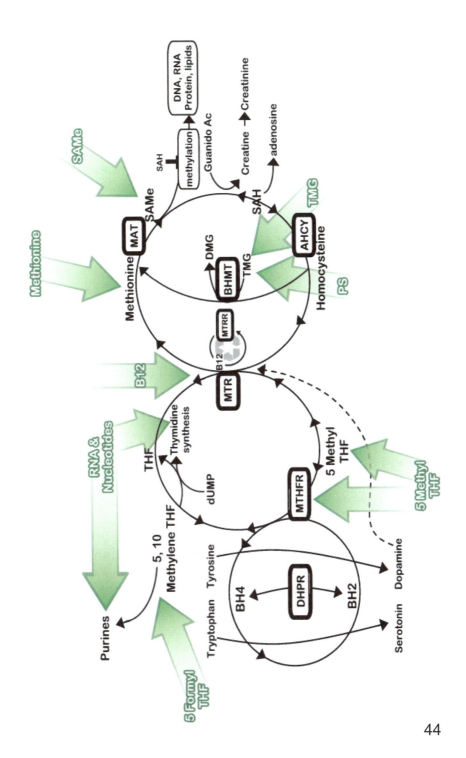

Descriptions of Specific Enzymes in the Pathway

I only believe in genetic testing if it gives you information that you can act on and do something positive with. I do not believe in testing just for the sake of testing. I actually think that genetic testing without any knowledge of how to address issues that are uncovered is unethical. My ultimate goal is to use the nutrigenomic testing as a guide to proper supplementation to bypass genetic weaknesses that are uncovered by SNP analysis.

It is important to understand that most mutations or variations that are uncovered are NOT "all or none mutations". In other words if you or your loved one has an MTHFR C677T mutation it does not mean that the MTHFR enzyme is completely "off". It means that it functions at lower efficiency. When you look at nutritional support, you are working to increase the ability of the methylation cycle to run properly; keeping in mind that it has been functioning to some degree.

This is a good opportunity to explain that a variation or a mutation does not always mean that an enzyme is not working at optimal efficiency. Rather it may *sometimes* mean that an enzyme is working at an increased level. The basic assumption is often made that if you see a mutation or a variation on a genetic test that the activity of the enzyme involved is decreased or impaired. However, changes in the DNA sequence can also result in increased activities of the enzymes involved. Additionally, changes in the DNA sequence can result in a lack of normal regulation of the enzyme involved.

There are several enzymatic mutations in the methylation pathway that have been described to occur that cause a decrease in the activity of the enzyme, such as the C677T mutation of the MTHFR gene. This mutation or variation, which can be identified by SNP analysis results in lowered enzyme activity and a subsequent increase in homocysteine levels as a result of the altered activity of this enzyme.

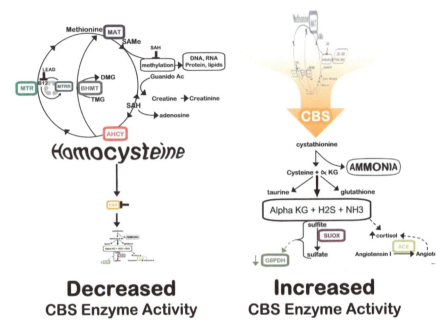

Decreased
CBS Enzyme Activity

Increased
CBS Enzyme Activity

Several other mutations in methylation pathway have been characterized which presumably result in increased activity of the relevant enzymes. According to reports in the literature, the C699T mutation of the cystathionine ß-synthase (CBS) results in increased enzymatic activity. This may explain the decreased levels of homocysteine seen in individuals that carry both the C677T MTHFR mutation as well as the C699T CBS mutation. Increased CBS enzyme activity would act to convert homocysteine more efficiently to cysteine, thereby lowering homocysteine levels. The increased activity of the CBS enzyme would serve to help to deplete the elevated levels of homocysteine that would be generated as a result of the C677T mutation in the MTHFR gene.

The A1298C mutation in the MTHFR enzyme represents an example of a variation in the regulatory region of an enzyme. The mutation in this case results in a change in the portion of the enzyme that binds to S adenosyl methionine (SAMe). The purported role of SAMe in binding to the MTHFR enzyme is to inhibit its function or down regulate MTHFR. This A1298C mutation may then result in an enzyme that is insensitive to inactivation or down regulation by SAMe. This would fit with the data that has found that individuals with the A1298C mutation do not show increased levels of homocysteine. This is in contrast to individuals with the C677T mutation that do show elevations in homocysteine levels.

While in vitro studies have found that the A1298C mutation does result in decreased enzyme activity, these studies were not conducted in the presence of SAMe. Without looking at enzyme activity in the presence of additional SAMe it would be impossible to determine if the effect of the A1298C mutation was to render the enzyme impervious to feedback inhibition by SAMe. If this is in fact the case it could result in a condition where the MTHFR enzyme would function with lowered efficiency but would not turn off in the presence of increased SAMe. The net result would be an enzyme that is always "ON"; this could result in a depletion of key intermediates in the methylation pathway in addition to secondary effects on enzyme function.

CBS : cystathionine ß-synthase
SUOX : sulfite oxidase

There are mutations in the CBS gene that impair its function. These mutations would lead to conditions in which homocysteine would be increased as a result of the inability of CBS to act appropriately in the transulfuration pathway There are also several mutations in the CBS enzyme that lead to increases in the enzymes activity. Both the CBS C699T as well as the CBS C1080T variations have been characterized as causing upregulations of enzyme activity.

Published information suggests that the CBS C699T mutation may result in a ten fold increase in enzyme activity as compared to the activity of the CBS without this mutation. This indicates how badly the pathway can be drained of its valuable intermediates by this upregulation, as well as the level of breakdown products that will be generated due to this mutation.

Increased CBS enzyme activity would act to convert homocysteine more efficiently to cysteine, thereby lowering homocysteine levels. Ultimately individuals with the CBS C699T up regulation of the CBS enzyme can generate more sulfur breakdown products with potential sulfur toxicity issues, enhanced ammonia production, and a lack of glutathione.

The level of cysteine helps to determine if glutathione or taurine is produced from the transulfuration reaction. High levels of cysteine favor the conversion of cysteine to sulfate and taurine rather than to glutathione. Consequently, the elevated rate of conversion of homocysteine to cysteine due to increased CBS activity would result in the subsequent conversion of cysteine to taurine and sulfate rather than to glutathione. While the temptation may be to add glutathione (due to low glutathione levels), this can potentially create additional issues due to sulfur excess in the body. The CBS upregulation is generating so many sulfur products that adding glutathione, another sulfur containing product, may be a problem for these individuals. Sensitivity to sulfur products and sulfur containing antibiotics is often symptomatic of this mutation.

The net effect of excess CBS activity is to take sulfur groups and nitrogen groups that are complexed in the methionine cycle and free them up. Having relatively free sulfur and nitrogen moieties has downstream consequences. Sulfur is able to directly activate the stress/cortisol response which can lead to elevations in adrenaline and depletion of dopamine and norepinephrine. A constant state of "flight or fight" as a result of chronic high levels of sulfur can also cause sympathetic versus parasympathetic overload. This cortisol response has a wide range of secondary effects in the body, including changes in magnesium/calcium, decreased levels of serotonin and dopamine, effects on the methylation cycle via phosphatidylserine levels, changes in gaba and glutamate as well as potentially depleting G6PDH and causing blood sugar issues.

Another possible consequence of the accelerated breakdown of homocysteine by an overactive CBS enzyme is that increased levels of alpha ketoglutarate will be generated in the body. Under ideal conditions, glutamine, glutamate, GABA and alpha keto glutarate can interconvert to form the intermediates that the body requires at any given time. However, aluminum and mercury inhibit some of the enzymes involved in these conversions. Aluminum inhibits the activity of glutamate dehydrogenase and mercury can inhibit the activity of glutamate synthase. GAD is the enzyme that converts glutamate to GABA, however its activity can be compromised by a wide range of mutations as well as the presence of auto antibodies against this enzyme.

Antibodies against GAD are seen in several viral and disease states. This combination of mutations, infectious diseases and toxic metals can create a possible scenario where excess alpha keto glutarate is being generated by breakdown of homocysteine but it cannot convert properly to form GABA. However this excess alpha KG can combine with the excess ammonia to form more glutamate. I have previously discussed at length the relationship between glutamate, excitotoxins and nerve damage.

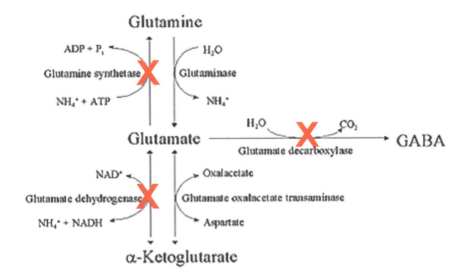

Individuals with CBS upregulations may not see high ammonia levels until they are supplementing the pathway to address other imbalances in this pathway. Other mutations in the methylation cycle can prevent the methylation pathway from functioning properly. Once the pathway is supplemented to function properly the intermediates of the cycle can be drained through the CBS enzyme activity into taurine, sulfur compounds and ammonia. Again, the reason you may not recognize this initially, is that other blocks in the pathway can mask the presence of this mutation until you supplement to bypass other mutations.

You may ask, why supplement at all then if it gives fuel for the CBS enzyme to generate products that are a problem for the body? The reason is that we need the methylation cycle for critical functions in the body. Methylation is needed to silence virus, to myelinate nerves, to make new T cells (so that we are not making auto antibodies, to respond properly to infectious agents and to reduce allergic inflammation), to make new DNA (i.e. to repair the gut lining), for neurotransmitters, for DNA regulation, detoxification of environmental toxins and the list goes on. It is critical to support any mutations in the methylation pathway so that it will function properly. However, for those individuals with CBS up regulations this is a "catch 22". As the pathway is supplemented you generate breakdown products that are a problem. Once you have supplemented with nutrients to bypass the CBS upregulation you are then in a better position to supplement the remainder of the methylation pathway for optimal function.

The sulfite oxidase enzyme (SUOX) is downstream from the CBS enzyme in this pathway. Molybdenum helps the body to process neurotoxic sulfite to sulfate via the enzyme sulfite oxidase. This reaction will be heavily taxed in individuals with CBS C699T upregulations and you will often see low levels of molybdenum in the body in spite of constant supplementation. If molybdenum is too low then the more toxic sulfite will not convert to the sulfate form.

By virtue of the fact that the methylation cycle is needed for synthesis of carnitine and COQ10, both important energy components of mitochondria, individuals with CBS mutations will likely be energy depleted. As a consequence of energy depletion, homocysteine produced is metabolized to alpha KG, NH3 (ammonia) and H2S (hydrogen sulfide). This suggests that another consequence of increased activity of the CBS enzyme is elevated levels of hydrogen sulfide in the brain.

Research has shown that hydrogen sulfide is able to induce a state of "tupor", or a state of semi hibernation. This may help to explain the "brain fog" that is often used to describe autistic children who carry the C699T+ mutations.

The impact of CBS upregulation mutations may have special implications for autism rates. Many have observed that the apparent rate of autism is increasing in this country and throughout the world.

As I have looked at genetic profiles for hundreds of children I have observed that the threshold for autism appears to have been lowered from a genetic standpoint. Thus far the genetics indicate that a majority of older autistic children carry the CBS C699T mutation. Younger children are presenting with autism carrying only mutations in MTR, MS_MTRR and MTHFR. The CBS C699T mutations are what I would call the "trump card". The CBS C699T mutations tend to over ride any other mutations as they can deplete all of the intermediates of the methionine pathway.

At one time it may have been necessary to have mutations like the CBS C699T that have a significant impact on the entire methylation pathway in order for autism to occur. Today, it appears that the bar has been lowered, and that "lesser" mutations are sufficient to cause autism. I believe this shift is due in part to the increase in heavy metal exposure from vaccines and the environment as well as the more intensive and accelerated vaccination program.

This may reflect the fact that the relative contributions of the factors that interact to cause multifactorial diseases may be different in every individual. There may be slight or enormous changes in the relative contributions of each of these components to disease. In the past the relative weight of the mutations in the pathway may have been heavier as compared to the weight of the environmental factors as components of the multifactorial disease of autism. Today, where the environmental factors may be a larger contributing component, it is possible that milder genetic components may be sufficient to cause autism. This shift then appears, and I emphasize appears, to have lowered the threshold for what mutations are necessary to predispose a child to autism.

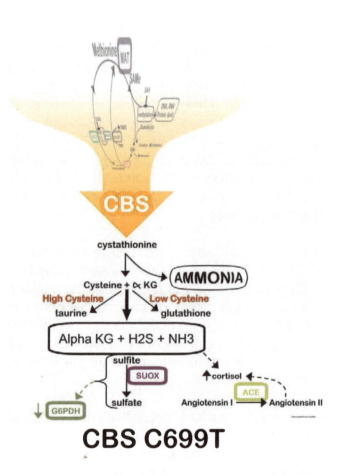

CBS C699T

MTR : methionine synthase
MTRR : methionine synthase reductase

Methionine synthase is responsible for the conversion of homocysteine back to methionine. A number of mutations that actually decrease the activity of this enzyme have been well characterized. Mutations that increase the activity have also been described for this gene. The A2756G mutation in the methionine synthase gene (MTR) has been reported to increase the activity of this enzyme.

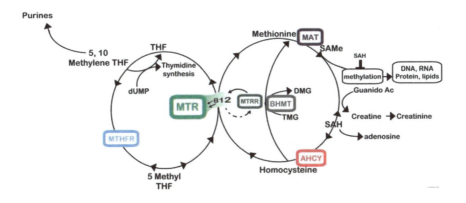

MTR A2756G

As is the case for the CBS C699T up regulation, the ultimate result of a number of these mutations that increase rather than decrease enzymatic activity is to deplete the methylation cycle of key intermediates that are needed for this pathway to function properly. In the case of the MTR A2756G, the net result of this upregulation may be to use up B12 at an even faster rate than normal, causing a depletion of methyl B12 from the cycle.

Decreased function of the MTR or a lack of B12 will diminish the level of conversion of homocysteine to methionine via this enzymatic route. A secondary route exists to convert homocysteine to methionine, utilizing the BHMT enzyme. Rather than using 5 methyl tetrahydrofolate and methyl B12 for this conversion, the BHMT enzyme utilizes TMG (betaine) as starting material for this alternative reaction. As described in the PDR (Physicians Desk Reference) *"Betaine or trimethylglycine is a quarternary ammonium compound that was first discovered in the juice of sugar beets (Beta vulgaris). Betaine is a metabolite of choline and is a substrate in one of the two recycling pathways that convert homocysteine to L-methionine. The other and principal recycling reaction is catalyzed by the enzyme methionine synthase and uses methylcobalamin as a cofactor and 5-methyltetrahydrofolate as a cosubstrate."*

Methionine synthase reductase (MTRR) acts in concert with methionine synthase enzyme to recycle homocysteine back to methionine. The function of methionine synthase reductase (MTRR) is to regenerate methyl B12 for methionine synthase to utilize. Mutations that impair the function of MTRR will have secondary consequences on the activity of the methionine synthase gene. Even if there are no

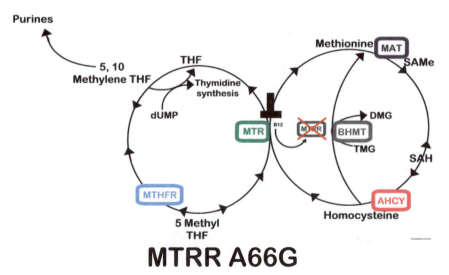

MTRR A66G

mutations in the methionine synthase gene, the inability of MTRR to regenerate sufficient methyl B12 will impact upon MTR activity in the methylation cycle.

The combination of a mutation in MTRR that compromises it's ability to regenerate B12, in concert with a MTR upregulation that is utilizing B12 at an accelerated rate would result in severely depleted levels of methyl B12 in the body. This would also create a roadblock in the methylation pathway between methionine and homocysteine that would require nutritional bypass for restored pathway function.

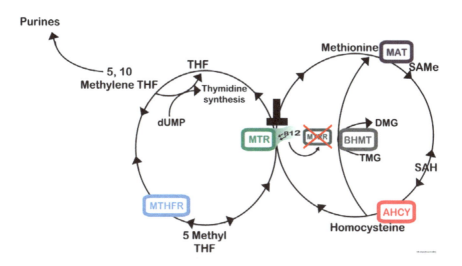

MTR A2756G / MTRR A66G Combination

COMT : catechol O methyl transferase
VDR : vitamin D receptor

If an individual has a COMT variation it means that they have a change in one of the amino acids of the enzyme. In the case of COMT one of the frequent amino acid changes is from a valine to a methionine. This is what is being tested for when the COMT V158M SNP test is run. The lab is able to look at the DNA to determine the information for which of these two amino acids that your copy of COMT contains. If you have the version with the information for a methionine in the sequence, it is written as COMT + meaning that you are positive for the methionine version. If you are COMT- it means that you do not have methionine in that spot of the enzyme and you have valine there instead. Since the valine in that spot is considered the "norm" the methionine represents the variation, so it is + for a variation being present.

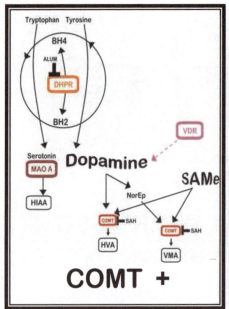

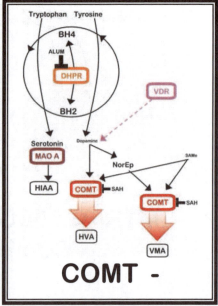

The form of the COMT with the variation (the methionine in it at a particular location) is a <u>less</u> efficient form of the enzyme. When the methionine is present it does not do as good a job of breaking down the dopamine. Therefore an individual who is COMT+ will not break dopamine down as easily. An individual who is COMT- (with the valine in that spot) will break dopamine down more efficiently.

The reason that the test results denote two ++ or two - - or + - is that we all have two copies of the DNA for the COMT enzyme; one from each parent.

The COMT enzyme uses methyl groups to help to inactivate dopamine. "COMT" stands for catechol O <u>methyl</u> transferase. So that when the COMT is working to inactivate dopamine and norepinephrine it does so by using methyl groups that you have available in your system. These methyl groups are donated by SAMe that is generated via the methylation pathway. Individuals who have the less efficient form of COMT (the COMT+ +) will be using less methyl groups because they are not inactivating dopamine as rapidly. Relative to the COMT - - individual they will have more methyl groups available for other reactions in the body.

I have found that both the COMT status, as well as the VDR Bsm and VDR Taq genes act in concert to have an impact upon overall need for methyl donors and dopamine support. In general individuals who are COMT - - will have lower levels of dopamine due to enhanced COMT activity and will need and are able to tolerate higher doses of methyl donors. Conversely individuals who are COMT + + will have increased levels of dopamine, due to less efficient breakdown, and need and tolerate lower amounts of methyl donors.

In addition, two of the three vitamin D receptor mutations also appear to play a role in dopamine levels and methyl donor tolerance. I believe that this is due to the relationship between vitamin D receptor and dopamine levels. Vitamin D increases the level of the enzyme involved in synthesizing dopamine. Increased levels of vitamin D would be expected to lead to increases in dopamine, norepinephrine and epinephrine. The VDR/Bsm – and VDR/Taq – genetic status results in higher levels of vitamin D. Therefore, individuals who are negative for the VDR Bsm and Taq polymorphisms (VDR Bsm/Taq - -) may have higher levels of dopamine due to enhanced levels of vitamin D. As would be expected if this were the case, I have found that these individuals are more sensitive to nutritional supplementation with methyl donors and nutrients that enhance dopamine levels than individuals who are homozygous (have both copies) for the VDR Bsm/Taq + + variation.

Increased levels of dopamine appear to aid in protecting cells from arsenic toxicity under conditions of low glutathione. This would suggest that supporting healthy dopamine levels for COMT – and VDR Bsm/Taq + individuals who also have glutathione mutations and/or CBS up regulations (which lead to decreased glutathione) may be helpful in reducing the effects of arsenic toxicity. Animal models indicate that chronic arsenic exposure leads to decreases in dopamine. Therefore low dopamine levels (in conjunction with reduced glutathione) create a "catch 22" whereby the toxicity of arsenic is increased, leading to further reductions in dopamine.

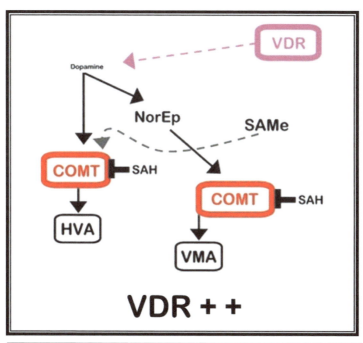

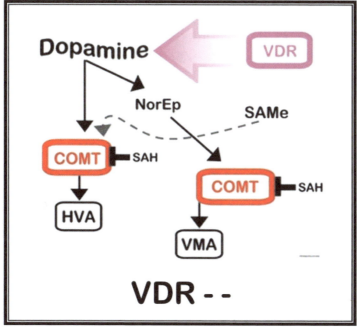

MTHFR :
methionine tetrahydrofolate reductase
DHPR : dihydropteridine reductase

The MTHFR enzyme is responsible for generating 5 methyl THF in the methylation pathway. The 5 methyl THF is needed to react with homocysteine to form methionine. The subsequent reaction to form methionine from 5 methyl THF and homocysteine is then the responsibility of the MTR/MTRR discussed above.

The C677 mutation in the MTHFR gene impacts the ability of the body to convert homocysteine to methionine. MTHFR C677T mutations in the MTHFR gene will therefore lead to increased levels of homocysteine if the body is not supplemented properly to address this mutation. High levels of homocysteine have been mentioned in association with heart disease, Alzheimer's disease as well as a range of inflammatory conditions. What this means is that individuals with the MTHFR C677T mutation are less able to make 5 methyl tetrahydrofolate and require supplementation with this form of folate to bypass this mutation.

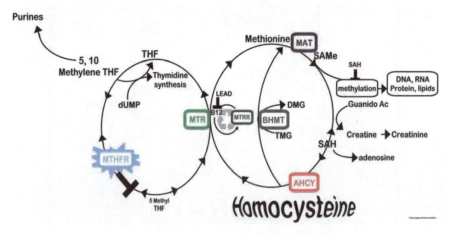

MTHFR C677T

There is literature to suggest that the MTHFR enzyme can function to facilitate more than one reaction. The C677T mutation in the MTHFR is a mutation in the forward reaction of this enzyme.

A second mutation in the MTHFR gene that has been well characterized is the A1298C mutation. The A1298C mutation has been mapped to the SAMe regulatory region of the gene. Mutations in the A1298C do <u>not</u> lead to increased levels of homocysteine; as such until now it has been felt that this mutation may not be of serious consequence.

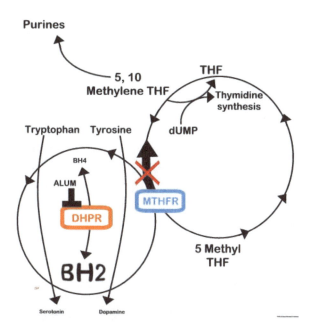

MTHFR A1298C

Literature suggests that in addition to the forward reaction that leads to 5methyl THF, that the MTHFR enzyme can drive a reverse reaction leading to formation of BH4 from BH2. I believe that the A1289C mutation is associated with a defect in this reverse reaction leading to the formation of BH4. If the reverse reaction is driven by SAMe binding to the regulatory site then the A1298C mutation would be associated with an inability to convert BH2 to BH4, and could result in exceedingly low BH4 levels.

This reaction, BH4 to BH2 is normally driven by the DHPR enzyme. However, this enzyme is inhibited by aluminum, mercury and lead. Toxic metal accumulation in the body is affected by the methylation pathway. As a consequence of impaired methylation cycle function, toxic metals can accumulate in the body that can decrease DHPR function and put more strain on the MTHFR driven pathway. If this hypothesis is correct, then individuals with MTHFR A1298C mutations could be seriously depleted in BH4. In addition there are a number of specific mutations that impair the function of the DHPR enzyme.

Low levels of BH4 are associated with more severe parasitic infections, diabetes as well as hypertension and arteriosclerosis. Serotonin synthesis, dopamine synthesis as well as ammonia detoxification require BH4. Factors that lead to more ammonia, such as high protein diets, and CBS C699T mutations generate elevated levels of ammonia that needs to be detoxified. Each molecule of ammonia requires two molecules of BH4 for ideal detoxification. It is clear to see how several of these factors may act together to impact ammonia detoxification as well as optimal BH4 levels for neurotransmitter synthesis. Keeping ammonia levels under control is of paramount importance for overall health and wellness, especially for an individual with MTHFR A1298C or DHPR mutations, as any excess ammonia generated can drain limited stores of BH4. Reductions in the reserves of BH4 will impact upon serotonin levels and dopamine levels.

BH4 appears to protect dopaminergic neurons from loss of glutathione. Under conditions of reduced glutathione (such as glutathione deficiency or CBS upregulations) these cells may require adequate levels of BH4 for survival. The combination of CBS C699T and MTHFR A1298C mutations may lead to both decreased glutathione as well as decreased BH4. This would leave dopaminergic neurons more susceptible to oxidative stress and environmental damage. Additional research suggests that BH4 is also able to protect GABA neurons from pathological conditions created by low glutathione levels.

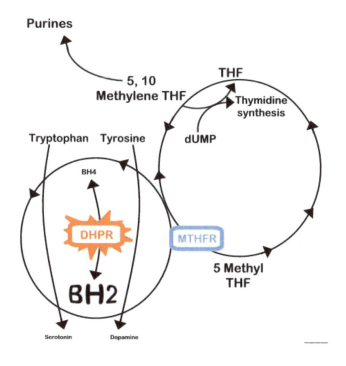

DHPR

OTC : ornithine transcarbamylase

The OTC enzyme is part of the urea cycle and is involved in the detoxification of ammonia. Mutations in the OTC gene can lead to elevations in ammonia levels. This increase in ammonia is via a distinctly different mechanism than the increases seen with CBS C699T mutations. A comprehensive OTC nutrigenomic screen is worth considering for those who show elevated ammonia levels and are negative for CBS upregulations. It is expected that combined mutations in OTC with CBS upregulations would result in extremely elevated ammonia levels.

OTC function can also be affected by the status of the methylation pathway. The region that turns on and off OTC function, the promoter region, is affected by methylation. Mutations that influence the ability of this region to be methylated have a profound effect on enzyme activity. As a consequence even if there is not a direct structural mutation in OTC, methylation cycle mutations can affect the function of this enzyme. Due to its overall effect on the methylation cycle, individuals with a CBS upregulation would likely have secondary issues with OTC function as a result of impaired methylation until supportive nutrition was used to bypass this mutation. Other mutations in the methylation pathway, such as MTR, MTRR, MTHFR would also be expected to have a negative impact on OTC function until proper nutritional supplementation was utilized to bypass these specific mutations.

Increased ammonia in the body can result as a function of an excessively high protein diet, CBS up regulations, OTC mutations, as well as decreased methylation which impairs OTC function. Increased entry of ammonia to the brain is a major cause of neurological disorders that are associated with hyperammonemia. It has been proposed that acute ammonia intoxification leads to increases in glutamate in the brain and activation of the NMDA receptor leading to excitotoxin damage as well as to seizure activity. Excess ammonia in the presence of calcium has also been shown to activate the mao A enzyme that breaks down serotonin. Consequences of elevated ammonia could then include excitotoxin damage and seizure activity as well as decreased levels of serotonin and dopamine.

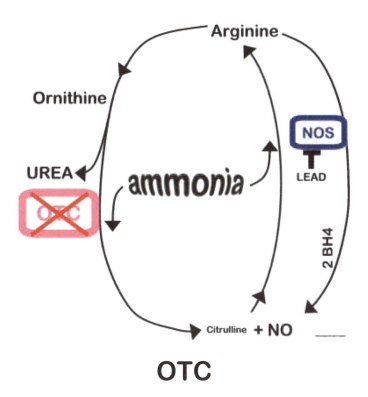

OTC

OTC mutations are an underlying risk factor for Reye's syndrome. Reye's syndrome occurs following a viral infection and the use of aspirin or other salicylates. It appears that the salicylates have a negative impact on mitochondrial energy production. (Recall that mutations in the methylation cycle also decrease components needed for mitochondrial energy). In susceptible individuals the effect of aspirin on the mitochondria leads to ammonia buildup and a drop in blood sugar levels. Individuals with mutations in the urea cycle have the greatest issue with Reye's syndrome.

Depletion of citrulline in the urea cycle as a result of OTC impairment can impact the ability of the Krebs cycle to function properly. The use of citrulline has been reported to be helpful as directly supporting the nutritional imbalance that is created as a result of an OTC mutation. In addition to supplementation with citrulline, the use of branched chain amino acids has been reported to be helpful in addressing OTC mutations. (The standard caveat for supplementing with BCAA holds here too, if the urine begins to smell like maple syrup discontinue the addition of BCAA immediately.) The BCAA may act to antagonize the effects of ammonia on serotonin levels, helping to balance serotonin levels.

The enzyme arginase is part of the final step of the urea cycle, generating urea and ornithine. Arginase is activated by manganese. In addition, manganese is involved in the production of dopamine as well as phosphatidylcholine and insulin. Obviously it is important to have sufficient levels of manganese in the body to activate arginase as well as for these other functions. While it is important to keep manganese levels in the normal range, excessive amounts of manganese can cause Parkinson like symptoms, so caution should be used with supplementation.

Part 2

Nutritional Analysis for Specific SNPs

This last section of the book is designed to give you suggestions for nutritional supplementation to bypass particular nutrigenomic profiles.

To use this section to your best advantage, look up your nutrigenomic profile, and then read about the supportive nutrients that may aid in bypassing the genetic weaknesses in your methylation pathway.

Please understand that I can only draw on my own experience in terms of supplement suggestions. As such I mention specific supplements that I have successfully used in my own personal practice. However, I have tried to explain my rationale for each choice so that others have the flexibility to make substitutions if they so choose.

Please note:

Supplements are not meant to treat or cure disease. In addition, supplementation suggestions are not meant to diagnose, treat or cure disease. This information is presented by an independent medical expert whose sources of information include studies from the world's medical and scientific literature, client records, and other clinical and anecdotal reports. All dosages suggested are based on the author's personal experiences. It is important to note that each person's body type and tolerance levels to supplements may be somewhat different. The publisher, author, and/or experts specifically cited in this publication are not responsible for any consequences, direct or indirect, resulting from any reader's action(s). This book is not intended to be a substitute for consultation with a health care provider. You, the reader are instructed to consult with your personal health care provider prior to acting on any suggestions contained in this book. The purpose of this publication is to educate the reader. The material in this book is for informational purposes only and is not intended for the diagnosis or treatment of disease.

General Mineral Support

- Mineral Support

As an introductory note, it is important to remember that as you support the methylation cycle in the body, it restores the body's natural ability to protect itself from chronic microbial infection as well as enhancing natural detoxification abilities. This can result in detoxification of virus, metals and bacteria that have accumulated in the body over time. This natural ability to detoxify is a separate function from active chelation therapy.

It is possible to use the following analogy to understand the distinction. You can think about the way the body handles toxins as a revolving door (the kind you see in office buildings or hotels). Toxins come in and toxins come out over the course of our lives. That is how most of us survive in a world filled with toxins. For individuals with methylation cycle mutations the revolving door is not working properly; toxins come in but they don't go out. Instead they accumulate. When you use a chelating agent, you are taking the toxins out the side door of the building. However the revolving door is still broken. Although the use of chelation can enhance the removal of toxins from the body, it cannot repair the revolving door. As a result toxins can still continue to accumulate in spite of chelation. Over time, especially if you stop chelating, you run the risk of toxins building up again unless you fix the broken door.

Running nutrigenomic tests help you to know what you need to do to fix the broken door so that it will work properly.

Regardless of whether you are using chelation therapy to speed up the detoxification process or simply supporting the methylation cycle to prevent health conditions that can occur as a result of methylation cycle mutations, using nutrition to bypass mutations can lead to detoxification of the body.

These are natural detoxification systems that operate on a regular basis for all of us, provided that our revolving door is functioning properly. For those whose revolving door is broken, once you do start to supplement for mutations you may find an increased level of detoxification from your system. This is especially true if your revolving door has been blocked for a long time. The use of urine, stool and blood toxic metal tests is one way to monitor the excretion of these metals and to verify that any symptoms you experience are related to natural detoxification. It is also important to monitor essential minerals in the body at the same time. I have noted that when we see excretion of heavy metals we often see a drop in essential minerals at the same time. This is why it is a good idea to follow essentials as well as toxic metals especially when you are seeing large amounts toxins on the toxic metal reports.

Excretion of mercury can affect the levels of lithium and iodine. It is possible to support iodine using 1/4 iodoral or other natural forms of iodine and to support healthy lithium levels with 1/4 lithium oratate. Decreases in calcium are often observed following the excretion of lead. Calcium can add to excitotoxin activity; consequently I prefer that calcium levels stay in the lower range of normal for those individuals with conditions that include elevated glutamate. If calcium support is needed I suggest utilizing herbs that include other components that may help to calm the body while increasing the level of calcium at the same time such as nettle, chamomile and chervil. If this is not sufficient to increase the levels within normal range then a supplement that includes calcium as well as magnesium and vitamins D and K is the preferred way to supplement. Calcium should be balanced by magnesium to help to prevent excitotoxin activity and vitamin D and K help to ensure the proper transport of calcium in the body. Chickweed, nettle, dandelion leaf and yellow dock are very nice natural sources of boron. The level of boron may drop along with calcium when you are excreting lead. Chickweed is also helpful for skin rashes, nettle helps to decrease inflammatory mediators and may also increase serotonin, dandelion leaf is supportive for the kidneys and yellow dock helps to support regular bowel movements. I prefer a mixture of small amounts of all of these to support boron if needed. However, I have listed some of the other benefits of these herbs to help you in choosing a single one from the list if needed.

There are a wide range of choices to support molybdenum and selenium. Healthy molybdenum levels are important to aid in sulfite detoxification and selenium is useful in binding to mercury. Magnesium can be supported as magnesium citrate, which is a very absorbable form and also will support citrate in the body or with a number of other products. Zinc can trigger activity at glutamate receptors in high doses. As a result I choose to keep zinc at 40mg per day or lower. I have supported zinc with zinc picolinate, the E lyte zinc, as well as zinc as a Krebs cycle intermediate. I prefer to keep magnesium levels higher than calcium so that the ratio favors more magnesium than calcium. Similarly I prefer that zinc levels exceed that of copper so that the relative ratio is in favor of zinc.

For overall general mineral support I often suggest BioNativus liquid minerals along with Cell food, using only two to three drops of each per day.

COMT - - VDR Bsm/Taq - -

- COMT - -   VDR Bsm/Taq - -

The nutrigenomics report for this individual shows no mutations in the COMT gene. This means that he/she is COMT- - so that he/she should be able to tolerate more methyl donors than individuals who are COMT ++. The COMT - - status indicates that he/she will break down dopamine more rapidly and as such will be depleting methyl groups from his/her methylation cycle in the process. However, this individual is also VDR Bsm/Taq - -. What this means in practical terms is that because he/she is COMT - - and VDR Bsm/Taq - - that he/she will behave more like a COMT + - individual even though he/she is COMT - -. While the use of supplements and foods to support optimal dopamine levels and methyl balance in the body is suggested, some additional caution should be exercised in the supplementation program to prevent mood swings from excess dopamine.

The COMT - - status, in spite of the VDR Bsm/Taq - - will have slowed down progress for optimal health and wellness. In addition, his/her toxic metal and viral burden may be higher than an individual who is COMT + + and VDR Bsm/Taq - -. As a result it may take a little longer to excrete all of the necessary metals and virus for optimal health.

It would make sense for this individual to eat a balance of high tryptophan foods and high tyrosine foods in an effort to support serotonin and dopamine levels. Tyrosine and tryptophan will compete with each other for transport into the cell. Tryptophan helps to support serotonin levels and tyrosine helps to support dopamine levels. Therefore if a balance of foods is used it will help to support healthy levels of both neurotransmitters. You can also consider the use of supplements to help to support healthy neurotransmitter levels. This would include using ¼ Mood S RNA once or twice per day and the use of St. John's Wort. This herb has some antiviral effects. In addition it is reported to help prevent the breakdown of serotonin. The use of small amounts of the Mood D and the Mood Focus RNA may be helpful to support healthy dopamine levels. Due to the COMT and VDR status, the suggested use is only 1/8 dropper per day. In addition to the Mood Focus and Mood D RNA consider supplementing with quercetin. This will help to support healthy dopamine levels and will help to limit allergic reactions in the body. Consider starting with 1/2 quercetin per day. Ginkgo has been reported to help to increase dopamine uptake; again the suggested starting point is ½ ginkgo per day. There is also a natural source of dopamine that is available that is an extract from Mucuna Pruriens. You could consider a very small sprinkle of this product however large doses are not suggested. Where he/she is VDR Bsm/Taq - - and COMT - - a benefit should be derived from low doses of supplements to support healthy dopamine levels as described above. However, if there are mood swings as a result of the supplements to support dopamine levels then you will want to decrease the dopamine supplements to half their initial dose in order to prevent future mood swings.

- COMT - - VDR Bsm/Taq - -
- MTR + or + +

There is a single mutation in the methionine synthase gene (MS or MTR). The methionine synthase mutation is an up regulation mutation that enhances the activity of the enzyme. This should cause the enzyme to use up added methyl B12 at an even faster rate than normal. What this means in practical terms is that he/she may be deficient in methyl B12. Due to his/her COMT and VDR Bsm/Taq status he/she should need and will tolerate the addition of methyl containing supplements. Supplementation with methyl B12 should be beneficial for him/her. This will both help to support the MTR mutation as well as to add methyl groups to his/her system. Supplementation can start with one chewable methyl B12 (5mg) daily. This can gradually be increased to two to three methyl B12 per day if he/she will tolerate it. If mood swings occur, then decrease the dose of methyl B12 back down to a more comfortable level. Literature suggests that oral B12 is as effective as injected B12; however as an alternative you can consider B12 injections. If you decide to use B12 injections it is preferable to use plain methyl B12 (no folinic or NAC). If you choose to use B12 injections it may be worth considering the addition of the chewable methyl B12 on the injections "off days". If you choose to use injections you can start with injections once a week and gradually increase to injections three times per week. This can be a very gradual process that is dictated by what he/she is able to tolerate; again using chewable B12 on the off days. If you decide to simply use the chewable methyl B12 this is an acceptable alternative. You may also want to add sublingual cyano B12 (once a day) to help to support his/her eyes.

There is a second pathway to the formation of methionine through the BHMT enzyme that will bypass this mutation in

the methionine synthase gene. This pathway uses phosphatidyl serine and /or TMG as donors for the reaction. It is wise to consider adding PS and a small amount of TMG to help to drive this reaction. While DMG works well to support language, it may be best to wait to add any DMG until this pathway is supplemented properly, as the DMG may be inhibiting this BHMT reaction to methionine. Supplementation for this part of the pathway also uses a low dose of TMG, choline and plain methionine. The HHC general vitamin is acceptable as a source for TMG, choline and methionine as well as the other general nutrients contained in it (½-1 in the morning and another ½-1 in the afternoon). In addition, phosphatidyl serine should also be added to help to support the "back door" reaction from homocysteine to methionine via the BHMT enzyme. Phosphatidyl serine is available as plain PS gel caps as well as a chewable form with DMAE (Pedi-Active). DMAE contains methyl groups so this is an ideal form for individuals who need extra methyl groups based on their COMT and VDR test results. Plain phosphatidyl serine is often available as a gel cap and this is a preferred form. Therefore if he/she will tolerate it, you should consider the use of one phosphatidyl serine gel cap as well as one of the chewable Pedi-Active PS with DMAE daily. This will help to support the alternative pathway that will bypass the mutation in the MTR gene.

Again, as with the methyl B12, if you find that this is more methyl groups than he/she can tolerate without causing mood swings, then eliminate the use of the Pedi-Active containing the DMAE.

To summarize at this point, due to the COMT - - status appropriate methylation supplementation would include: ¼ Folapro, ¼ Intrinsic B12, methyl B12, ¼ nucleotides, SAMe (1/2 to one per day), ¼ dropper methylation support RNA, one plain phosphatidyl serine gel cap, one Pedi-Active chewable

phosphatidyl serine with DMAE, and one to two of the HHC neurological health general vitamins daily. SAMe is a critical intermediate in numerous reactions in the body. SAMe is a sulfur containing compound that is a critical intermediate in the methylation methionine/folate cycle and also serves as a methyl donor in the body. In the future you should consider the use of other methyl donors. You may want to consider the use of curcumin, melatonin, FgF, theanine, ZEN, and MSM (not for those with CBS C699T + status) in addition to the specific methyl donors already listed (SAMe, methyl B12).

As the level of B12 becomes more in balance following appropriate supplementation to address the methylation cycle mutation it will also help in balancing glutamate and GABA levels. In addition GABA can be added directly. Where he/she is COMT - - he/she should also be able to tolerate, and benefit from ZEN which contains theanine in addition to GABA, as theanine has methyl groups. There are several other supplements that are very useful for balancing glutamate and GABA; these include taurine, pycnogenol and grape seed extract. These three are included in the general vitamin; however you may want to consider adding in additional amounts of pycnogenol, grape seed extract and taurine (except for no additional taurine for those with a CBS C699T+ mutation) as needed based on behavior especially as there are only very low doses of these in the general vitamin. GABA levels are related to language, as well as to anxiety levels, particularly anxiety in response to low blood sugar.

Lead inhibits a critical enzyme in the pathway for heme synthesis. A block in this pathway creates a build up of an intermediate that competes with GABA. Reduced GABA activity can cause auditory processing issues as well as language problems, and anxiety. In addition, inhibition of this pathway by lead can cause anemia, as well as the inability to make groups that are needed for B12 synthesis. A lack of

these groups will exacerbate mutations in methionine synthase and methionine synthase reductase. This again points to the need for added B12 for individuals with mutations in this portion of the methylation cycle as well as the use of supplements to address lead toxicity in the body. The use of weekly baths in Beyond Clean, which contains EDTA should help to address lead toxicity in a very gentle manner that is suitable to most systems. It is also valuable to consider the use of ½ EDTA capsule per day or the use of EDTA chewing gum.

Once the methylation cycle is supplemented properly you may begin to see an increased level of detoxification. Generally there will be a one week "honeymoon" period followed by a regression in behaviors as the creatinine starts to climb. In order to monitor this and to understand changes in behavior that may occur as a result of this detoxification, it is a good idea to take spot urine samples and run urine toxic metal tests. It may seem like a supplement is non ideal for an individual. However, it is difficult to tell the difference between a negative reaction to a supplement and the behavioral impact of detoxification or a mood swing due to dopamine fluxes as the methylation pathway is supplemented properly; that is why use of regular urine toxic metal tests is so critical. The urine samples will help to separate the effects of methylation support on detoxification from supplements that do not agree with an individual.

- COMT - -   VDR Bsm/Taq - -
- MTRR + or + +

    There is also a mutation in the methionine synthase reductase gene (MS_MTRR or MSR). What this means in practical terms is that he/she may be deficient in methyl B12. The function of MSR is to regenerate B12 for the methionine synthase to utilize. Due to his/her COMT and VDR Bsm/Taq status he/she should need and will tolerate the addition of methyl containing supplements. Supplementation with methyl B12 should be beneficial for him/her. This will both help to support the MTR mutation as well as to add methyl groups to his/her system. Supplementation can start with one chewable methyl B12 (5mg) daily. This can gradually be increased to two to three methyl B12 per day if he/she will tolerate it. If mood swings occur, then decrease the dose of methyl B12 back down to a more comfortable level. Literature suggests that oral B12 is as effective as injected B12; however as an alternative you can consider B12 injections. If you decide to use B12 injections it is preferable to use plain methyl B12 (no folinic or NAC). If you choose to use B12 injections it may be worth considering the addition of the chewable methyl B12 on the injections "off days". If you choose to use injections you can start with injections once a week and gradually increase to injections three times per week. This can be a very gradual process that is dictated by what he/she is able to tolerate; again using chewable B12 on the off days. If you decide to simply use the chewable methyl B12 this is an acceptable alternative. You may also want to add sublingual cyano B12 (once a day) to help to support his/her eyes.

    There is a second pathway to the formation of methionine through the BHMT enzyme that will bypass this mutation in the methionine synthase reductase gene. This pathway uses phosphatidyl serine and /or TMG as donors for the reaction. It

is wise to consider adding PS and a small amount of TMG to help to drive this reaction. While DMG works well to support language, it may be best to wait to add any DMG until this pathway is supplemented properly, as the DMG may be inhibiting this BHMT reaction to methionine. Supplementation for this part of the pathway also uses a low dose of TMG, choline and plain methionine. The HHC general vitamin is acceptable as a source for TMG, choline and methionine as well as the other general nutrients contained in it (½-1 in the morning and another ½-1 in the afternoon). In addition, phosphatidyl serine should also be added to help to support the "back door" reaction from homocysteine to methionine via the BHMT enzyme. Phosphatidyl serine is available as plain PS gel caps as well as a chewable form with DMAE (Pedi-Active). DMAE contains methyl groups so this is an ideal form for individuals who need extra methyl groups based on their COMT and VDR test results. Plain phosphatidyl serine is often available as a gel cap and this is a preferred form. Therefore if he/she will tolerate it, you should consider the use of one phosphatidyl serine gel cap as well as one of the chewable Pedi-Active PS with DMAE daily. This will help to support the alternative pathway that will bypass the mutation in the MTR gene.

Again, as with the methyl B12, if you find that this is more methyl groups than he/she can tolerate without causing mood swings, then eliminate the use of the Pedi-Active containing the DMAE.

To summarize at this point, due to the COMT + - status appropriate methylation supplementation would include: ¼ Folapro, ¼ Intrinsic B12, methyl B12, ¼ nucleotides, SAMe (1/2 to one per day), ¼ dropper methylation support RNA, one plain phosphatidyl serine gel cap, one Pedi-Active chewable phosphatidyl serine with DMAE, and one to two of the HHC neurological health general vitamins daily. SAMe is a critical intermediate in numerous reactions in the body. SAMe is a sulfur containing compound that is a critical intermediate in the methylation methionine/folate cycle and also serves as a methyl donor in the body. If this is more methylation than he/she is able to handle, and he/she begins to exhibit mood swings, then you can adjust the balance between the use of methyl and hydroxy B12 to favor more hydroxy B12, and also decrease the dose of SAMe or eliminate it entirely. Conversely, in the future if he/she is tolerating methyl donors well, you can consider the use of other methyl donors. You may want to consider the use of curcumin, melatonin, FgF, theanine, ZEN, and MSM (not for those with CBS C699T + status) in addition to the specific methyl donors already listed (SAMe, methyl B12).

As the level of B12 becomes more in balance following appropriate supplementation to address the methylation cycle mutation it will also help in balancing glutamate and GABA levels. In addition GABA can be added directly. Plain GABA will be tolerated due to the COMT and VDR status. Where he/she is COMT + - he/she should also be able to tolerate, and benefit from low doses of ZEN which contains theanine in addition to GABA, as theanine has methyl groups. There are several other supplements that are very useful for balancing glutamate and GABA; these include taurine, pycnogenol and grape seed extract. These three are included in the general vitamin; however you may want to consider adding in additional amounts of pycnogenol, grape seed extract and taurine (except for no additional taurine for those with a CBS C699T+ mutation) as needed based on behavior especially as there are only very low doses of these in the general vitamin. GABA levels are related to language, as well as to anxiety levels, particularly anxiety in response to low blood sugar.

Lead inhibits a critical enzyme in the pathway for heme synthesis. A block in this pathway creates a build up of an

intermediate that competes with GABA. Reduced GABA activity can cause auditory processing issues as well as language problems, and anxiety. In addition, inhibition of this pathway by lead can cause anemia, as well as the inability to make groups that are needed for B12 synthesis. A lack of these groups will exacerbate mutations in methionine synthase and methionine synthase reductase. This again points to the need for added B12 for individuals with mutations in this portion of the methylation cycle as well as the use of supplements to address lead toxicity in the body. The use of weekly baths in Beyond Clean, which contains EDTA should help to address lead toxicity in a very gentle manner that is suitable to most systems. It is also valuable to consider the use of ½ EDTA capsule per day or the use of EDTA chewing gum.

Once the methylation cycle is supplemented properly you may begin to see an increased level of detoxification. Generally there will be a one week "honeymoon" period followed by a regression in behaviors as the creatinine starts to climb. In order to monitor this and to understand changes in behavior that may occur as a result of this detoxification, it is a good idea to take spot urine samples and run urine toxic metal tests. It may seem like a supplement is non ideal for an individual. However, it is difficult to tell the difference between a negative reaction to a supplement and the behavioral impact of detoxification or a mood swing due to dopamine fluxes as the methylation pathway is supplemented properly; that is why use of regular urine toxic metal tests is so critical. The urine samples will help to separate the effects of methylation support on detoxification from supplements that do not agree with an individual.

- COMT - - VDR Bsm/Taq - -
- MTR + or + +
- MTRR + or + +

There is also a mutation in the methionine synthase reductase gene (MS_MTRR or MSR), as well as a mutation in the methionine synthase gene (MS or MTR). The function of MSR is to regenerate B12 for the MS to utilize. The methionine synthase mutation is an up regulation mutation that enhances the activity of the enzyme. This should cause the enzyme to use up added B12 at an even faster rate than normal. What this means in practical terms is that he/she may be severely deficient in methyl B12. The supplementation of B12 is therefore very important for him/her. Due to his/her COMT and VDR Bsm/Taq status he/she should need and will tolerate the addition of methyl containing supplements. Supplementation with methyl B12 should be beneficial for him/her. This will both help to support the MTR mutation as well as to add methyl groups to his/her system. Supplementation can start with one chewable methyl B12 (5mg) daily. This can gradually be increased to two to three methyl B12 per day if he/she will tolerate it. If mood swings occur, then decrease the dose of methyl B12 back down to a more comfortable level. Literature suggests that oral B12 is as effective as injected B12; however as an alternative you can consider B12 injections. If you decide to use B12 injections it is preferable to use plain methyl B12 (no folinic or NAC). If you choose to use B12 injections it may be worth considering the addition of the chewable methyl B12 on the injections "off days". If you choose to use injections you can start with injections once a week and gradually increase to injections three times per week. This can be a very gradual process that is dictated by what he/she is able to tolerate; again using chewable B12 on the off days. If you decide to simply use the chewable methyl B12 this is an acceptable alternative. You

may also want to add sublingual cyano B12 (once a day) to help to support his/her eyes.

There is a second pathway to the formation of methionine through the BHMT enzyme that will bypass both of these mutations in the methionine synthase reductase and the methionine synthase genes. This pathway uses phosphatidyl serine and /or TMG as donors for the reaction. It is wise to consider adding PS and a small amount of TMG to help to drive this reaction. While DMG works well to support language, it may be best to wait to add any DMG until this pathway is supplemented properly, as the DMG may be inhibiting this BHMT reaction to methionine. Supplementation for this part of the pathway also uses a low dose of TMG, choline and plain methionine. The HHC general vitamin is acceptable as a source for TMG, choline and methionine as well as the other general nutrients contained in it (½-1 in the morning and another ½-1 in the afternoon). In addition, phosphatidyl serine should also be added to help to support the "back door" reaction from homocysteine to methionine via the BHMT enzyme. Phosphatidyl serine is available as plain PS gel caps as well as a chewable form with DMAE (Pedi-Active). DMAE contains methyl groups so this is an ideal form for individuals who need extra methyl groups based on their COMT and VDR test results. Plain phosphatidyl serine is often available as a gelcap and this is a preferred form. Therefore if he/she will tolerate it, you should consider the use of one phosphatidyl serine gelcap as well as one of the chewable Pedi-Active PS with DMAE daily. This will help to support the alternative pathway that will bypass the mutations in the MTR and MS_MTRR genes.

Again, as with the methyl B12, if you find that this is more methyl groups than he/she can tolerate without causing mood swings, then eliminate the use of the Pedi-Active containing the DMAE.

To summarize at this point, due to the COMT + - status appropriate methylation supplementation would include: ¼ Folapro, ¼ Intrinsic B12, methyl B12, ¼ nucleotides, SAMe (1/2 to one per day), ¼ dropper methylation support RNA, one plain phosphatidyl serine gel cap, one Pedi-Active chewable phosphatidyl serine with DMAE, and one to two of the HHC neurological health general vitamins daily. SAMe is a critical intermediate in numerous reactions in the body. SAMe is a sulfur containing compound that is a critical intermediate in the methylation methionine/folate cycle and also serves as a methyl donor in the body. If this is more methylation than he/she is able to handle, and he/she begins to exhibit mood swings, then you can adjust the balance between the use of methyl and hydroxy B12 to favor more hydroxy B12, and also decrease the dose of SAMe or eliminate it entirely. Conversely, in the future if he/she is tolerating methyl donors well, you can consider the use of other methyl donors. You may want to consider the use of curcumin, melatonin, FgF, theanine, ZEN, and MSM (not for those with CBS C699T + status) in addition to the specific methyl donors already listed (SAMe, methyl B12).

As the level of B12 becomes more in balance following appropriate supplementation to address the methylation cycle mutation it will also help in balancing glutamate and GABA levels. In addition GABA can be added directly. Plain GABA will be tolerated due to the COMT and VDR status. Where he/she is COMT + - he/she should also be able to tolerate, and benefit from low doses of ZEN which contains theanine in addition to GABA, as theanine has methyl groups. There are several other supplements that are very useful for balancing glutamate and GABA; these include taurine, pycnogenol and grape seed extract. These three are included in the general vitamin; however you may want to consider adding in additional amounts of pycnogenol, grape seed extract and taurine (except for <u>no</u> additional taurine for those with a CBS

C699T+ mutation) as needed based on behavior especially as there are only very low doses of these in the general vitamin. GABA levels are related to language, as well as to anxiety levels, particularly anxiety in response to low blood sugar.

Lead inhibits a critical enzyme in the pathway for heme synthesis. A block in this pathway creates a build up of an intermediate that competes with GABA. Reduced GABA activity can cause auditory processing issues as well as language problems, and anxiety. In addition, inhibition of this pathway by lead can cause anemia, as well as the inability to make groups that are needed for B12 synthesis. A lack of these groups will exacerbate mutations in methionine synthase and methionine synthase reductase. This again points to the need for added B12 for individuals with mutations in this portion of the methylation cycle as well as the use of supplements to address lead toxicity in the body. The use of weekly baths in Beyond Clean, which contains EDTA should help to address lead toxicity in a very gentle manner that is suitable to most systems. It is also valuable to consider the use of ½ EDTA capsule per day or the use of EDTA chewing gum.

Once the methylation cycle is supplemented properly you may begin to see an increased level of detoxification. Generally there will be a one week "honeymoon" period followed by a regression in behaviors as the creatinine starts to climb. In order to monitor this and to understand changes in behavior that may occur as a result of this detoxification, it is a good idea to take spot urine samples and run urine toxic metal tests. It may seem like a supplement is non ideal for an individual. However, it is difficult to tell the difference between a negative reaction to a supplement and the behavioral impact of detoxification or a mood swing due to dopamine fluxes as the methylation pathway is supplemented properly; that is why use of regular urine toxic metal tests is so critical. The urine samples will help to separate the effects of methylation support on detoxification from supplements that do not agree with an individual.

COMT - -   VDR Bsm/Taq + -

- COMT - -   VDR BsmTaq + -

The nutrigenomics report for this individual shows no mutations in the COMT gene. This means that he/she is COMT- - so that he/she should be able to tolerate more methyl donors than individuals who are COMT ++. The COMT - - status indicates that he/she will break down dopamine more rapidly and as such will be depleting methyl groups from his/her methylation cycle in the process. However, this individual is also VDR Bsm/Taq + -. What this means in practical terms is that because he/she is COMT - - and heterozygous for the VDR Bsm/Taq (+ -) that to a certain extent he/she will behave more like a COMT + - individual even though he/she is COMT - -. While the use of supplements and foods to support optimal dopamine levels and methyl balance in the body is suggested, some caution should be exercised in the supplementation program to prevent mood swings from excess dopamine.

The COMT - - status, in spite of the VDR Bsm/Taq + - will have slowed down progress for optimal health and wellness. In addition, his/her toxic metal and viral burden may be higher than an individual who is COMT + + and VDR Bsm/Taq - -. As a result it may take a little longer to excrete all of the necessary metals and virus for optimal health.

It would make sense for this individual to eat a balance of high tryptophan foods and high tyrosine foods in an effort to support serotonin and dopamine levels. Tyrosine and tryptophan will compete with each other for transport into the cell. Tryptophan helps to support serotonin levels and tyrosine helps to support dopamine levels. Therefore if a balance of foods is used it will help to support healthy levels of both neurotransmitters. You can also consider the use of supplements to help to support healthy neurotransmitter levels. This would include using ¼ Mood S RNA once or twice per day and the use of St. John's Wort. This herb has some antiviral effects. In addition it is reported to help prevent the breakdown of serotonin. The use of small amounts of the Mood D and the Mood Focus RNA may be helpful to support healthy dopamine levels. Due to the COMT + - status, the suggested use is only 1/8 dropper per day. In addition to the Mood Focus and Mood D RNA consider supplementing with quercetin. This will help to support healthy dopamine levels and will help to limit allergic reactions in the body. Consider starting with 1/2 quercetin per day. Ginkgo has been reported to help to increase dopamine uptake; again the suggested starting point is ½ ginkgo per day. There is also a natural source of dopamine that is available that is an extract from Mucuna Pruriens. You could consider a very small sprinkle of this product however large doses are not suggested. Where he/she is VDR Bsm/Taq + - and COMT - - a benefit should be derived from low doses of supplements to support healthy dopamine levels as described above. However, if there are mood swings as a result of the supplements to support dopamine levels then you will want to decrease the dopamine supplements to half their initial dose in order to prevent future mood swings.

- COMT - - VDR Bsm/Taq + -
- MTRR + or + +

There is also a mutation in the methionine synthase reductase gene (MS_MTRR or MSR). What this means in practical terms is that he/she may be deficient in methyl B12. The function of MSR is to regenerate B12 for the methionine synthase to utilize. Due to his/her COMT and VDR Bsm/Taq status he/she should need and will tolerate the addition of methyl containing supplements. Supplementation with methyl B12 should be beneficial for him/her. This will both help to support the MTR mutation as well as to add methyl groups to his/her system. Supplementation can start with one chewable methyl B12 (5mg) daily. This can gradually be increased to two to three methyl B12 per day if he/she will tolerate it. If mood swings occur, then decrease the dose of methyl B12 back down to a more comfortable level. Literature suggests that oral B12 is as effective as injected B12; however as an alternative you can consider B12 injections. If you decide to use B12 injections it is preferable to use plain methyl B12 (no folinic or NAC). If you choose to use B12 injections it may be worth considering the addition of the chewable methyl B12 on the injections "off days". If you choose to use injections you can start with injections once a week and gradually increase to injections three times per week. This can be a very gradual process that is dictated by what he/she is able to tolerate; again using chewable B12 on the off days. If you decide to simply use the chewable methyl B12 this is an acceptable alternative. You may also want to add sublingual cyano B12 (once a day) to help to support his/her eyes.

There is a second pathway to the formation of methionine through the BHMT enzyme that will bypass this mutation in the methionine synthase reductase gene. This pathway uses phosphatidyl serine and /or TMG as donors for the reaction. It

is wise to consider adding PS and a small amount of TMG to help to drive this reaction. While DMG works well to support language, it may be best to wait to add any DMG until this pathway is supplemented properly, as the DMG may be inhibiting this BHMT reaction to methionine. Supplementation for this part of the pathway also uses a low dose of TMG, choline and plain methionine. The HHC general vitamin is acceptable as a source for TMG, choline and methionine as well as the other general nutrients contained in it (½-1 in the morning and another ½-1 in the afternoon). In addition, phosphatidyl serine should also be added to help to support the "back door" reaction from homocysteine to methionine via the BHMT enzyme. Phosphatidyl serine is available as plain PS gel caps as well as a chewable form with DMAE (Pedi-Active). DMAE contains methyl groups so this is an ideal form for individuals who need extra methyl groups based on their COMT and VDR test results. Plain phosphatidyl serine is often available as a gelcap and this is a preferred form. Therefore if he/she will tolerate it, you should consider the use of one phosphatidyl serine gelcap as well as one of the chewable Pedi-Active PS with DMAE daily. This will help to support the alternative pathway that will bypass the mutation in the MTR gene.

Again, as with the methyl B12, if you find that this is more methyl groups than he/she can tolerate without causing mood swings, then eliminate the use of the Pedi-Active containing the DMAE.

To summarize at this point, due to the COMT - - status appropriate methylation supplementation would include: ¼ Folapro, ¼ Intrinsic B12, methyl B12, ¼ nucleotides, SAMe (1/2 to one per day), ¼ dropper methylation support RNA, one plain phosphatidyl serine gel cap, one Pedi-Active chewable phosphatidyl serine with DMAE, and one to two of the HHC neurological health general vitamins daily. SAMe is a critical intermediate in numerous reactions in the body. SAMe is a sulfur containing compound that is a critical intermediate in the methylation methionine/folate cycle and also serves as a methyl donor in the body. In the future you should consider the use of other methyl donors. You may want to consider the use of curcumin, melatonin, FgF, theanine, ZEN, and MSM (not for those with CBS C699T + status) in addition to the specific methyl donors already listed (SAMe, methyl B12).

As the level of B12 becomes more in balance following appropriate supplementation to address the methylation cycle mutation it will also help in balancing glutamate and GABA levels. In addition GABA can be added directly. Where he/she is COMT - - he/she should also be able to tolerate, and benefit from ZEN which contains theanine in addition to GABA, as theanine has methyl groups. There are several other supplements that are very useful for balancing glutamate and GABA; these include taurine, pycnogenol and grape seed extract. These three are included in the general vitamin; however you may want to consider adding in additional amounts of pycnogenol, grape seed extract and taurine (except for no additional taurine for those with a CBS C699T+ mutation) as needed based on behavior especially as there are only very low doses of these in the general vitamin. GABA levels are related to language, as well as to anxiety levels, particularly anxiety in response to low blood sugar.

Lead inhibits a critical enzyme in the pathway for heme synthesis. A block in this pathway creates a build up of an intermediate that competes with GABA. Reduced GABA activity can cause auditory processing issues as well as language problems, and anxiety. In addition, inhibition of this pathway by lead can cause anemia, as well as the inability to make groups that are needed for B12 synthesis. A lack of these groups will exacerbate mutations in methionine synthase and methionine synthase reductase. This again points to the need for added B12 for individuals with mutations in this portion of the methylation cycle as well as the use of supplements to address lead toxicity in the body. The use of weekly baths in Beyond Clean, which contains EDTA should help to address lead toxicity in a very gentle manner that is suitable to most systems. It is also valuable to consider the use of ½ EDTA capsule per day or the use of EDTA chewing gum.

Once the methylation cycle is supplemented properly you may begin to see an increased level of detoxification. Generally there will be a one week "honeymoon" period followed by a regression in behaviors as the creatinine starts to climb. In order to monitor this and to understand changes in behavior that may occur as a result of this detoxification, it is a good idea to take spot urine samples and run urine toxic metal tests. It may seem like a supplement is non ideal for an individual. However, it is difficult to tell the difference between a negative reaction to a supplement and the behavioral impact of detoxification or a mood swing due to dopamine fluxes as the methylation pathway is supplemented properly; that is why use of regular urine toxic metal tests is so critical. The urine samples will help to separate the effects of methylation support on detoxification from supplements that do not agree with an individual.

- COMT - - VDR Bsm/Taq +-
- MTR + or + +

There is a single mutation in the methionine synthase gene (MS or MTR). The methionine synthase mutation is an up regulation mutation that enhances the activity of the enzyme. This should cause the enzyme to use up added methyl B12 at an even faster rate than normal. What this means in practical terms is that he/she may be deficient in methyl B12. Due to his/her COMT and VDR Bsm/Taq status he/she should need and will tolerate the addition of methyl containing supplements. Supplementation with methyl B12 should be beneficial for him/her. This will both help to support the MTR mutation as well as to add methyl groups to his/her system. Supplementation can start with one chewable methyl B12 (5mg) daily. This can gradually be increased to two to three methyl B12 per day if he/she will tolerate it. If mood swings occur, then decrease the dose of methyl B12 back down to a more comfortable level. Literature suggests that oral B12 is as effective as injected B12; however as an alternative you can consider B12 injections. If you decide to use B12 injections it is preferable to use plain methyl B12 (no folinic or NAC). If you choose to use B12 injections it may be worth considering the addition of the chewable methyl B12 on the injections "off days". If you choose to use injections you can start with injections once a week and gradually increase to injections three times per week. This can be a very gradual process that is dictated by what he/she is able to tolerate; again using chewable B12 on the off days. If you decide to simply use the chewable methyl B12 this is an acceptable alternative. You may also want to add sublingual cyano B12 (once a day) to help to support his/her eyes.

There is a second pathway to the formation of methionine through the BHMT enzyme that will bypass this mutation in

the methionine synthase gene. This pathway uses phosphatidyl serine and /or TMG as donors for the reaction. It is wise to consider adding PS and a small amount of TMG to help to drive this reaction. While DMG works well to support language, it may be best to wait to add any DMG until this pathway is supplemented properly, as the DMG may be inhibiting this BHMT reaction to methionine. Supplementation for this part of the pathway also uses a low dose of TMG, choline and plain methionine. The HHC general vitamin is acceptable as a source for TMG, choline and methionine as well as the other general nutrients contained in it (½-1 in the morning and another ½-1 in the afternoon). In addition, phosphatidyl serine should also be added to help to support the "back door" reaction from homocysteine to methionine via the BHMT enzyme. Phosphatidyl serine is available as plain PS gel caps as well as a chewable form with DMAE (Pedi-Active). DMAE contains methyl groups so this is an ideal form for individuals who need extra methyl groups based on their COMT and VDR test results. Plain phosphatidyl serine is often available as a gelcap and this is a preferred form. Therefore if he/she will tolerate it, you should consider the use of one phosphatidyl serine gelcap as well as one of the chewable Pedi-Active PS with DMAE daily. This will help to support the alternative pathway that will bypass the mutation in the MTR gene.

Again, as with the methyl B12, if you find that this is more methyl groups than he/she can tolerate without causing mood swings, then eliminate the use of the Pedi-Active containing the DMAE.

To summarize at this point, due to the COMT - - status appropriate methylation supplementation would include: ¼ Folapro, ¼ Intrinsic B12, methyl B12, ¼ nucleotides, SAMe (1/2 to one per day), ¼ dropper methylation support RNA, one plain phosphatidyl serine gel cap, one Pedi-Active chewable

phosphatidyl serine with DMAE, and one to two of the HHC neurological health general vitamins daily. SAMe is a critical intermediate in numerous reactions in the body. SAMe is a sulfur containing compound that is a critical intermediate in the methylation methionine/folate cycle and also serves as a methyl donor in the body. In the future you should consider the use of other methyl donors. You may want to consider the use of curcumin, melatonin, FgF, theanine, ZEN, and MSM (not for those with CBS C699T + status) in addition to the specific methyl donors already listed (SAMe, methyl B12).

As the level of B12 becomes more in balance following appropriate supplementation to address the methylation cycle mutation it will also help in balancing glutamate and GABA levels. In addition GABA can be added directly. Where he/she is COMT - - he/she should also be able to tolerate, and benefit from ZEN which contains theanine in addition to GABA, as theanine has methyl groups. There are several other supplements that are very useful for balancing glutamate and GABA; these include taurine, pycnogenol and grape seed extract. These three are included in the general vitamin; however you may want to consider adding in additional amounts of pycnogenol, grape seed extract and taurine (except for no additional taurine for those with a CBS C699T+ mutation) as needed based on behavior especially as there are only very low doses of these in the general vitamin. GABA levels are related to language, as well as to anxiety levels, particularly anxiety in response to low blood sugar.

Lead inhibits a critical enzyme in the pathway for heme synthesis. A block in this pathway creates a build up of an intermediate that competes with GABA. Reduced GABA activity can cause auditory processing issues as well as language problems, and anxiety. In addition, inhibition of this pathway by lead can cause anemia, as well as the inability to make groups that are needed for B12 synthesis. A lack of

these groups will exacerbate mutations in methionine synthase and methionine synthase reductase. This again points to the need for added B12 for individuals with mutations in this portion of the methylation cycle as well as the use of supplements to address lead toxicity in the body. The use of weekly baths in Beyond Clean, which contains EDTA should help to address lead toxicity in a very gentle manner that is suitable to most systems. It is also valuable to consider the use of ½ EDTA capsule per day or the use of EDTA chewing gum.

Once the methylation cycle is supplemented properly you may begin to see an increased level of detoxification. Generally there will be a one week "honeymoon" period followed by a regression in behaviors as the creatinine starts to climb. In order to monitor this and to understand changes in behavior that may occur as a result of this detoxification, it is a good idea to take spot urine samples and run urine toxic metal tests. It may seem like a supplement is non ideal for an individual. However, it is difficult to tell the difference between a negative reaction to a supplement and the behavioral impact of detoxification or a mood swing due to dopamine fluxes as the methylation pathway is supplemented properly; that is why use of regular urine toxic metal tests is so critical. The urine samples will help to separate the effects of methylation support on detoxification from supplements that do not agree with an individual.

- COMT - - VDR Bsm/Taq + -
- MTR + or + +
- MTRR + or + +

There is also a mutation in the methionine synthase reductase gene (MS_MTRR or MSR), as well as a mutation in the methionine synthase gene (MS or MTR). The function of MSR is to regenerate B12 for the MS to utilize. The methionine synthase mutation is an up regulation mutation that enhances the activity of the enzyme. This should cause the enzyme to use up added B12 at an even faster rate than normal. What this means in practical terms is that he/she may be severely deficient in methyl B12. The supplementation of B12 is therefore very important for him/her. Due to his/her COMT and VDR Bsm/Taq status he/she should need and will tolerate the addition of methyl containing supplements. Supplementation with methyl B12 should be beneficial for him/her. This will both help to support the MTR mutation as well as to add methyl groups to his/her system. Supplementation can start with one chewable methyl B12 (5mg) daily. This can gradually be increased to two to three methyl B12 per day if he/she will tolerate it. If mood swings occur, then decrease the dose of methyl B12 back down to a more comfortable level. Literature suggests that oral B12 is as effective as injected B12; however as an alternative you can consider B12 injections. If you decide to use B12 injections it is preferable to use plain methyl B12 (no folinic or NAC). If you choose to use B12 injections it may be worth considering the addition of the chewable methyl B12 on the injections "off days". If you choose to use injections you can start with injections once a week and gradually increase to injections three times per week. This can be a very gradual process that is dictated by what he/she is able to tolerate; again using chewable B12 on the off days. If you decide to simply use the chewable methyl B12 this is an acceptable alternative. You

may also want to add sublingual cyano B12 (once a day) to help to support his/her eyes.

There is a second pathway to the formation of methionine through the BHMT enzyme that will bypass both of these mutations in the methionine synthase reductase and the methionine synthase genes. This pathway uses phosphatidyl serine and /or TMG as donors for the reaction. It is wise to consider adding PS and a small amount of TMG to help to drive this reaction. While DMG works well to support language, it may be best to wait to add any DMG until this pathway is supplemented properly, as the DMG may be inhibiting this BHMT reaction to methionine. Supplementation for this part of the pathway also uses a low dose of TMG, choline and plain methionine. The HHC general vitamin is acceptable as a source for TMG, choline and methionine as well as the other general nutrients contained in it (½-1 in the morning and another ½-1 in the afternoon). In addition, phosphatidyl serine should also be added to help to support the "back door" reaction from homocysteine to methionine via the BHMT enzyme. Phosphatidyl serine is available as plain PS gel caps as well as a chewable form with DMAE (Pedi-Active). DMAE contains methyl groups so this is an ideal form for individuals who need extra methyl groups based on their COMT and VDR test results. Plain phosphatidyl serine is often available as a gel cap and this is a preferred form. Therefore if he/she will tolerate it, you should consider the use of one phosphatidyl serine gel cap as well as one of the chewable Pedi-Active PS with DMAE daily. This will help to support the alternative pathway that will bypass the mutations in the MTR and MS_MTRR genes.

Again, as with the methyl B12, if you find that this is more methyl groups than he/she can tolerate without causing mood swings, then eliminate the use of the Pedi-Active containing the DMAE.

To summarize at this point, due to the COMT - - status appropriate methylation supplementation would include: ¼ Folapro, ¼ Intrinsic B12, methyl B12, ¼ nucleotides, SAMe (1/2 to one per day), ¼ dropper methylation support RNA, one plain phosphatidyl serine gel cap, one Pedi-Active chewable phosphatidyl serine with DMAE, and one to two of the HHC neurological health general vitamins daily. SAMe is a critical intermediate in numerous reactions in the body. SAMe is a sulfur containing compound that is a critical intermediate in the methylation methionine/folate cycle and also serves as a methyl donor in the body. In the future you should consider the use of other methyl donors. You may want to consider the use of curcumin, melatonin, FgF, theanine, ZEN, and MSM (not for those with CBS C699T + status) in addition to the specific methyl donors already listed (SAMe, methyl B12).

As the level of B12 becomes more in balance following appropriate supplementation to address the methylation cycle mutation it will also help in balancing glutamate and GABA levels. In addition GABA can be added directly. Where he/she is COMT - - he/she should also be able to tolerate, and benefit from ZEN which contains theanine in addition to GABA, as theanine has methyl groups. There are several other supplements that are very useful for balancing glutamate and GABA; these include taurine, pycnogenol and grape seed extract. These three are included in the general vitamin; however you may want to consider adding in additional amounts of pycnogenol, grape seed extract and taurine (except for no additional taurine for those with a CBS C699T+ mutation) as needed based on behavior especially as there are only very low doses of these in the general vitamin. GABA levels are related to language, as well as to anxiety levels, particularly anxiety in response to low blood sugar.

Lead inhibits a critical enzyme in the pathway for heme synthesis. A block in this pathway creates a build up of an

intermediate that competes with GABA. Reduced GABA activity can cause auditory processing issues as well as language problems, and anxiety. In addition, inhibition of this pathway by lead can cause anemia, as well as the inability to make groups that are needed for B12 synthesis. A lack of these groups will exacerbate mutations in methionine synthase and methionine synthase reductase. This again points to the need for added B12 for individuals with mutations in this portion of the methylation cycle as well as the use of supplements to address lead toxicity in the body. The use of weekly baths in Beyond Clean, which contains EDTA should help to address lead toxicity in a very gentle manner that is suitable to most systems. It is also valuable to consider the use of ½ EDTA capsule per day or the use of EDTA chewing gum.

Once the methylation cycle is supplemented properly you may begin to see an increased level of detoxification. Generally there will be a one week "honeymoon" period followed by a regression in behaviors as the creatinine starts to climb. In order to monitor this and to understand changes in behavior that may occur as a result of this detoxification, it is a good idea to take spot urine samples and run urine toxic metal tests. It may seem like a supplement is non ideal for an individual. However, it is difficult to tell the difference between a negative reaction to a supplement and the behavioral impact of detoxification or a mood swing due to dopamine fluxes as the methylation pathway is supplemented properly; that is why use of regular urine toxic metal tests is so critical. The urine samples will help to separate the effects of methylation support on detoxification from supplements that do not agree with an individual.

COMT - - VDR Bsm/Taq + +

- COMT - -   VDR Bsm/Taq + +

The nutrigenomics report for this individual shows no mutations in the COMT gene. This means that he/she is COMT- - so that he/she should be able to tolerate, and will need more methyl donors than individuals who are COMT + +. In addition he/she is also homozygous for the VDR Bsm/Taq (+ +) as a result he/she may have particularly low levels of dopamine and will benefit from added methyl donors and other supplements to support healthy dopamine levels and for methyl balance in the body. In addition, his/her toxic metal and viral burden may be higher than an individuals who is COMT + + and VDR Bsm/Taq - -. As a result it may take a little longer to excrete all of the necessary metals and virus for optimal health.

It would make sense for this individual to eat a balance of high tryptophan foods and high tyrosine foods in an effort to support serotonin and dopamine levels. Tyrosine and tryptophan will compete with each other for transport into the cell. Tryptophan helps to support serotonin levels and tyrosine helps to support dopamine levels. Therefore if a balance of foods is used it will help to support healthy levels of both neurotransmitters. You can also consider the use of supplements to help to support healthy neurotransmitter levels. This would include using ¼ Mood S RNA once or twice per day and the use of St. John's Wort. This herb has some antiviral effects. In addition it is reported to help prevent the breakdown of serotonin. The use of small amounts of the Mood D and the Mood Focus RNA may be helpful to support healthy dopamine levels. Due to the COMT + - status, the suggested use is only 1/8 dropper per day. In addition to the Mood Focus and Mood D RNA consider supplementing with quercetin. This will help to support healthy dopamine levels and will help to limit allergic reactions in the body. Consider starting with 1/2 quercetin per day. Ginkgo has been reported to help to increase dopamine uptake; again the suggested starting point is ½ ginkgo per day. There is also a natural source of dopamine that is available that is an extract from Mucuna Pruriens. You could consider a small sprinkle of this product but I would not suggest large doses.

- COMT - - VDR Bsm/Taq + +
- MTR + or + +

There is a single mutation in the methionine synthase gene (MS or MTR). The methionine synthase mutation is an up regulation mutation that enhances the activity of the enzyme. This should cause the enzyme to use up added methyl B12 at an even faster rate than normal. What this means in practical terms is that he/she may be deficient in methyl B12. Due to his/her COMT and VDR Bsm/Taq status he/she should need and will tolerate the addition of methyl containing supplements. Supplementation with methyl B12 should be beneficial for him/her. This will both help to support the MTR mutation as well as to add methyl groups to his/her system. Supplementation can start with one chewable methyl B12 (5mg) daily. This can gradually be increased to two to three methyl B12 per day if he/she will tolerate it. If mood swings occur, then decrease the dose of methyl B12 back down to a more comfortable level. Literature suggests that oral B12 is as effective as injected B12; however as an alternative you can consider B12 injections. If you decide to use B12 injections it is preferable to use plain methyl B12 (no folinic or NAC). If you choose to use B12 injections it may be worth considering the addition of the chewable methyl B12 on the injections "off days". If you choose to use injections you can start with injections once a week and gradually increase to injections three times per week. This can be a very gradual process that is dictated by what he/she is able to tolerate; again using chewable B12 on the off days. If you decide to simply use the chewable methyl B12 this is an acceptable alternative. You may also want to add sublingual cyano B12 (once a day) to help to support his/her eyes.

There is a second pathway to the formation of methionine through the BHMT enzyme that will bypass this mutation in

the methionine synthase gene. This pathway uses phosphatidyl serine and /or TMG as donors for the reaction. It is wise to consider adding PS and a small amount of TMG to help to drive this reaction. While DMG works well to support language, it may be best to wait to add any DMG until this pathway is supplemented properly, as the DMG may be inhibiting this BHMT reaction to methionine. Supplementation for this part of the pathway also uses a low dose of TMG, choline and plain methionine. The HHC general vitamin is acceptable as a source for TMG, choline and methionine as well as the other general nutrients contained in it (½-1 in the morning and another ½-1 in the afternoon). In addition, phosphatidyl serine should also be added to help to support the "back door" reaction from homocysteine to methionine via the BHMT enzyme. Phosphatidyl serine is available as plain PS gel caps as well as a chewable form with DMAE (Pedi-Active). DMAE contains methyl groups so this is an ideal form for individuals who need extra methyl groups based on their COMT and VDR test results. Plain phosphatidyl serine is often available as a gel cap and this is a preferred form. Therefore if he/she will tolerate it, you should consider the use of one phosphatidyl serine gel cap as well as one of the chewable Pedi-Active PS with DMAE daily. This will help to support the alternative pathway that will bypass the mutation in the MTR gene.

Again, as with the methyl B12, if you find that this is more methyl groups than he/she can tolerate without causing mood swings, then eliminate the use of the Pedi-Active containing the DMAE.

To summarize at this point, due to the COMT - - status appropriate methylation supplementation would include: ¼ Folapro, ¼ Intrinsic B12, methyl B12, ¼ nucleotides, SAMe (1/2 to one per day), ¼ dropper methylation support RNA, one plain phosphatidyl serine gel cap, one Pedi-Active chewable

phosphatidyl serine with DMAE, and one to two of the HHC neurological health general vitamins daily. SAMe is a critical intermediate in numerous reactions in the body. SAMe is a sulfur containing compound that is a critical intermediate in the methylation methionine/folate cycle and also serves as a methyl donor in the body. In the future you should consider the use of other methyl donors. You may want to consider the use of curcumin, melatonin, FgF, theanine, ZEN, and MSM (not for those with CBS C699T + status) in addition to the specific methyl donors already listed (SAMe, methyl B12).

As the level of B12 becomes more in balance following appropriate supplementation to address the methylation cycle mutation it will also help in balancing glutamate and GABA levels. In addition GABA can be added directly. Where he/she is COMT - - he/she should also be able to tolerate, and benefit from ZEN which contains theanine in addition to GABA, as theanine has methyl groups. There are several other supplements that are very useful for balancing glutamate and GABA; these include taurine, pycnogenol and grape seed extract. These three are included in the general vitamin; however you may want to consider adding in additional amounts of pycnogenol, grape seed extract and taurine (except for no additional taurine for those with a CBS C699T+ mutation) as needed based on behavior especially as there are only very low doses of these in the general vitamin. GABA levels are related to language, as well as to anxiety levels, particularly anxiety in response to low blood sugar.

Lead inhibits a critical enzyme in the pathway for heme synthesis. A block in this pathway creates a build up of an intermediate that competes with GABA. Reduced GABA activity can cause auditory processing issues as well as language problems, and anxiety. In addition, inhibition of this pathway by lead can cause anemia, as well as the inability to make groups that are needed for B12 synthesis. A lack of

these groups will exacerbate mutations in methionine synthase and methionine synthase reductase. This again points to the need for added B12 for individuals with mutations in this portion of the methylation cycle as well as the use of supplements to address lead toxicity in the body. The use of weekly baths in Beyond Clean, which contains EDTA should help to address lead toxicity in a very gentle manner that is suitable to most systems. It is also valuable to consider the use of ½ EDTA capsule per day or the use of EDTA chewing gum.

Once the methylation cycle is supplemented properly you may begin to see an increased level of detoxification. Generally there will be a one week "honeymoon" period followed by a regression in behaviors as the creatinine starts to climb. In order to monitor this and to understand changes in behavior that may occur as a result of this detoxification, it is a good idea to take spot urine samples and run urine toxic metal tests. It may seem like a supplement is non ideal for an individual. However, it is difficult to tell the difference between a negative reaction to a supplement and the behavioral impact of detoxification or a mood swing due to dopamine fluxes as the methylation pathway is supplemented properly; that is why use of regular urine toxic metal tests is so critical. The urine samples will help to separate the effects of methylation support on detoxification from supplements that do not agree with an individual.

- COMT - - VDR Bsm/Taq + +
- MTRR + or + +

There is also a mutation in the methionine synthase reductase gene (MS_MTRR or MSR). What this means in practical terms is that he/she may be deficient in methyl B12. The function of MSR is to regenerate B12 for the methionine synthase to utilize. Due to his/her COMT and VDR Bsm/Taq status he/she should need and will tolerate the addition of methyl containing supplements. Supplementation with methyl B12 should be beneficial for him/her. This will both help to support the MTR mutation as well as to add methyl groups to his/her system. Supplementation can start with one chewable methyl B12 (5mg) daily. This can gradually be increased to two to three methyl B12 per day if he/she will tolerate it. If mood swings occur, then decrease the dose of methyl B12 back down to a more comfortable level. Literature suggests that oral B12 is as effective as injected B12; however as an alternative you can consider B12 injections. If you decide to use B12 injections it is preferable to use plain methyl B12 (no folinic or NAC). If you choose to use B12 injections it may be worth considering the addition of the chewable methyl B12 on the injections "off days". If you choose to use injections you can start with injections once a week and gradually increase to injections three times per week. This can be a very gradual process that is dictated by what he/she is able to tolerate; again using chewable B12 on the off days. If you decide to simply use the chewable methyl B12 this is an acceptable alternative. You may also want to add sublingual cyano B12 (once a day) to help to support his/her eyes.

There is a second pathway to the formation of methionine through the BHMT enzyme that will bypass this mutation in the methionine synthase reductase gene. This pathway uses phosphatidyl serine and /or TMG as donors for the reaction. It

is wise to consider adding PS and a small amount of TMG to help to drive this reaction. While DMG works well to support language, it may be best to wait to add any DMG until this pathway is supplemented properly, as the DMG may be inhibiting this BHMT reaction to methionine. Supplementation for this part of the pathway also uses a low dose of TMG, choline and plain methionine. The HHC general vitamin is acceptable as a source for TMG, choline and methionine as well as the other general nutrients contained in it (½-1 in the morning and another ½-1 in the afternoon). In addition, phosphatidyl serine should also be added to help to support the "back door" reaction from homocysteine to methionine via the BHMT enzyme. Phosphatidyl serine is available as plain PS gel caps as well as a chewable form with DMAE (Pedi-Active). DMAE contains methyl groups so this is an ideal form for individuals who need extra methyl groups based on their COMT and VDR test results. Plain phosphatidyl serine is often available as a gelcap and this is a preferred form. Therefore if he/she will tolerate it, you should consider the use of one phosphatidyl serine gelcap as well as one of the chewable Pedi-Active PS with DMAE daily. This will help to support the alternative pathway that will bypass the mutation in the MTR gene.

Again, as with the methyl B12, if you find that this is more methyl groups than he/she can tolerate without causing mood swings, then eliminate the use of the Pedi-Active containing the DMAE.

To summarize at this point, due to the COMT - - status appropriate methylation supplementation would include: ¼ Folapro, ¼ Intrinsic B12, methyl B12, ¼ nucleotides, SAMe (1/2 to one per day), ¼ dropper methylation support RNA, one plain phosphatidyl serine gel cap, one Pedi-Active chewable phosphatidyl serine with DMAE, and one to two of the HHC neurological health general vitamins daily. SAMe is a critical intermediate in numerous reactions in the body. SAMe is a sulfur containing compound that is a critical intermediate in the methylation methionine/folate cycle and also serves as a methyl donor in the body. In the future you should consider the use of other methyl donors. You may want to consider the use of curcumin, melatonin, FgF, theanine, ZEN, and MSM (not for those with CBS C699T + status) in addition to the specific methyl donors already listed (SAMe, methyl B12).

As the level of B12 becomes more in balance following appropriate supplementation to address the methylation cycle mutation it will also help in balancing glutamate and GABA levels. In addition GABA can be added directly. Where he/she is COMT - - he/she should also be able to tolerate, and benefit from ZEN which contains theanine in addition to GABA, as theanine has methyl groups. There are several other supplements that are very useful for balancing glutamate and GABA; these include taurine, pycnogenol and grape seed extract. These three are included in the general vitamin; however you may want to consider adding in additional amounts of pycnogenol, grape seed extract and taurine (except for _no_ additional taurine for those with a CBS C699T+ mutation) as needed based on behavior especially as there are only very low doses of these in the general vitamin. GABA levels are related to language, as well as to anxiety levels, particularly anxiety in response to low blood sugar.

Lead inhibits a critical enzyme in the pathway for heme synthesis. A block in this pathway creates a build up of an intermediate that competes with GABA. Reduced GABA activity can cause auditory processing issues as well as language problems, and anxiety. In addition, inhibition of this pathway by lead can cause anemia, as well as the inability to make groups that are needed for B12 synthesis. A lack of these groups will exacerbate mutations in methionine synthase and methionine synthase reductase. This again points to the need for added B12 for individuals with mutations in this portion of the methylation cycle as well as the use of supplements to address lead toxicity in the body. The use of weekly baths in Beyond Clean, which contains EDTA should help to address lead toxicity in a very gentle manner that is suitable to most systems. It is also valuable to consider the use of ½ EDTA capsule per day or the use of EDTA chewing gum.

Once the methylation cycle is supplemented properly you may begin to see an increased level of detoxification. Generally there will be a one week "honeymoon" period followed by a regression in behaviors as the creatinine starts to climb. In order to monitor this and to understand changes in behavior that may occur as a result of this detoxification, it is a good idea to take spot urine samples and run urine toxic metal tests. It may seem like a supplement is non ideal for an individual. However, it is difficult to tell the difference between a negative reaction to a supplement and the behavioral impact of detoxification or a mood swing due to dopamine fluxes as the methylation pathway is supplemented properly; that is why use of regular urine toxic metal tests is so critical. The urine samples will help to separate the effects of methylation support on detoxification from supplements that do not agree with an individual.

- COMT - - VDR Bsm/Taq + +
- MTR + or + +
- MTRR + or + +

There is also a mutation in the methionine synthase reductase gene (MS_MTRR or MSR), as well as a mutation in the methionine synthase gene (MS or MTR). The function of MSR is to regenerate B12 for the MS to utilize. The methionine synthase mutation is an up regulation mutation that enhances the activity of the enzyme. This should cause the enzyme to use up added B12 at an even faster rate than normal. What this means in practical terms is that he/she may be severely deficient in methyl B12. The supplementation of B12 is therefore very important for him/her. Due to his/her COMT and VDR Bsm/Taq status he/she should need and will tolerate the addition of methyl containing supplements. Supplementation with methyl B12 should be beneficial for him/her. This will both help to support the MTR mutation as well as to add methyl groups to his/her system. Supplementation can start with one chewable methyl B12 (5mg) daily. This can gradually be increased to two to three methyl B12 per day if he/she will tolerate it. If mood swings occur, then decrease the dose of methyl B12 back down to a more comfortable level. Literature suggests that oral B12 is as effective as injected B12; however as an alternative you can consider B12 injections. If you decide to use B12 injections it is preferable to use plain methyl B12 (no folinic or NAC). If you choose to use B12 injections it may be worth considering the addition of the chewable methyl B12 on the injections "off days". If you choose to use injections you can start with injections once a week and gradually increase to injections three times per week. This can be a very gradual process that is dictated by what he/she is able to tolerate; again using chewable B12 on the off days. If you decide to simply use the chewable methyl B12 this is an acceptable alternative. You

may also want to add sublingual cyano B12 (once a day) to help to support his/her eyes.

There is a second pathway to the formation of methionine through the BHMT enzyme that will bypass both of these mutations in the methionine synthase reductase and the methionine synthase genes. This pathway uses phosphatidyl serine and /or TMG as donors for the reaction. It is wise to consider adding PS and a small amount of TMG to help to drive this reaction. While DMG works well to support language, it may be best to wait to add any DMG until this pathway is supplemented properly, as the DMG may be inhibiting this BHMT reaction to methionine. Supplementation for this part of the pathway also uses a low dose of TMG, choline and plain methionine. The HHC general vitamin is acceptable as a source for TMG, choline and methionine as well as the other general nutrients contained in it (½-1 in the morning and another ½-1 in the afternoon). In addition, phosphatidyl serine should also be added to help to support the "back door" reaction from homocysteine to methionine via the BHMT enzyme. Phosphatidyl serine is available as plain PS gel caps as well as a chewable form with DMAE (Pedi-Active). DMAE contains methyl groups so this is an ideal form for individuals who need extra methyl groups based on their COMT and VDR test results. Plain phosphatidyl serine is often available as a gel cap and this is a preferred form. Therefore if he/she will tolerate it, you should consider the use of one phosphatidyl serine gel cap as well as one of the chewable Pedi-Active PS with DMAE daily. This will help to support the alternative pathway that will bypass the mutations in the MTR and MS_MTRR genes.

Again, as with the methyl B12, if you find that this is more methyl groups than he/she can tolerate without causing mood swings, then eliminate the use of the Pedi-Active containing the DMAE.

To summarize at this point, due to the COMT - - status appropriate methylation supplementation would include: ¼ Folapro, ¼ Intrinsic B12, methyl B12, ¼ nucleotides, SAMe (1/2 to one per day), ¼ dropper methylation support RNA, one plain phosphatidyl serine gel cap, one Pedi-Active chewable phosphatidyl serine with DMAE, and one to two of the HHC neurological health general vitamins daily. SAMe is a critical intermediate in numerous reactions in the body. SAMe is a sulfur containing compound that is a critical intermediate in the methylation methionine/folate cycle and also serves as a methyl donor in the body. In the future you should consider the use of other methyl donors. You may want to consider the use of curcumin, melatonin, FgF, theanine, ZEN, and MSM (not for those with CBS C699T + status) in addition to the specific methyl donors already listed (SAMe, methyl B12).

As the level of B12 becomes more in balance following appropriate supplementation to address the methylation cycle mutation it will also help in balancing glutamate and GABA levels. In addition GABA can be added directly. Where he/she is COMT - - he/she should also be able to tolerate, and benefit from ZEN which contains theanine in addition to GABA, as theanine has methyl groups. There are several other supplements that are very useful for balancing glutamate and GABA; these include taurine, pycnogenol and grape seed extract. These three are included in the general vitamin; however you may want to consider adding in additional amounts of pycnogenol, grape seed extract and taurine (except for no additional taurine for those with a CBS C699T+ mutation) as needed based on behavior especially as there are only very low doses of these in the general vitamin. GABA levels are related to language, as well as to anxiety levels, particularly anxiety in response to low blood sugar.

Lead inhibits a critical enzyme in the pathway for heme synthesis. A block in this pathway creates a build up of an

intermediate that competes with GABA. Reduced GABA activity can cause auditory processing issues as well as language problems, and anxiety. In addition, inhibition of this pathway by lead can cause anemia, as well as the inability to make groups that are needed for B12 synthesis. A lack of these groups will exacerbate mutations in methionine synthase and methionine synthase reductase. This again points to the need for added B12 for individuals with mutations in this portion of the methylation cycle as well as the use of supplements to address lead toxicity in the body. The use of weekly baths in Beyond Clean, which contains EDTA should help to address lead toxicity in a very gentle manner that is suitable to most systems. It is also valuable to consider the use of ½ EDTA capsule per day or the use of EDTA chewing gum.

Once the methylation cycle is supplemented properly you may begin to see an increased level of detoxification. Generally there will be a one week "honeymoon" period followed by a regression in behaviors as the creatinine starts to climb. In order to monitor this and to understand changes in behavior that may occur as a result of this detoxification, it is a good idea to take spot urine samples and run urine toxic metal tests. It may seem like a supplement is non ideal for an individual. However, it is difficult to tell the difference between a negative reaction to a supplement and the behavioral impact of detoxification or a mood swing due to dopamine fluxes as the methylation pathway is supplemented properly; that is why use of regular urine toxic metal tests is so critical. The urine samples will help to separate the effects of methylation support on detoxification from supplements that do not agree with an individual.

COMT + - VDR Bsm/Taq - -

- COMT + -   VDR Bsm/Taq - -

The nutrigenomics report for this individual shows a single mutation in the COMT gene. This means that he/she is COMT+ - so that they should be able to tolerate more methyl donors than individuals who are COMT + +, however it will still be important to watch the total number of methyl donors that are used in supplements as he/she is also VDR Bsm/Taq - -. What this means in practical terms is that because he/she is COMT + - and VDR Bsm/Taq + - , he/she will behave like a COMT + + individual in terms of their responses to most methyl donors and will be particularly sensitive to added methyl donors. This will mean that supporting dopamine levels should not be an issue as we look at the overall supplement plan. However, the COMT + - status, as compared to a COMT + + indicates that he/she will still be able to break down dopamine more rapidly than a COMT + + individual and as such will still be depleting methyl groups from their methylation cycle in the process. What this means in practical terms is that because he/she is COMT + - and VDR Bsm/Taq + - you will be able to use a few more methyl donors in key places in his/her supplement program. However, please use caution in the use of methyl donors and pay careful attention to the total amount of methyl donors in the supplement plan as well as to the total amount of dopamine containing foods that are ingested on a given day. Too many methyl donors may cause he/she to have mood swings. Pay careful attention to lithium and iodine levels during any detoxification of heavy metals, as excretion of mercury can affect the levels of lithium and iodine. These essential minerals appear to play an important role in helping to balance mood swings that can occur as a result of dopamine fluxes. These dopamine fluxes are much more of an issue in individuals who are COMT + - /VDR Bsm and Taq - -, than in those who are COMT - - and VDR / Bsm and Taq + +.

It is also important to pay attention to foods containing a high level of tyrosine that may increase dopamine levels. Tyrosine and tryptophan will compete with each other for transport into the cell. Tryptophan helps to support serotonin levels and tyrosine helps to support dopamine levels. Therefore it is wise to consider the list of high tryptophan and high dopamine foods and try to concentrate on more of the high tryptophan foods and to limit the intake of the high tyrosine foods in an effort to support serotonin levels and to prevent mood swings due to dopamine overload.

- COMT + - VDR Bsm/Taq - -
- MTRR + or + +

There is a mutation in the methionine synthase reductase gene (MS_MTRR or MSR). The methionine synthase mutation is an up regulation mutation that enhances the activity of the enzyme. This should cause the enzyme to use up added B12 at an even faster rate than normal. What this means in practical terms is that he/she may be deficient in methyl B12. The supplementation of B12 is therefore very important for him/her. What will be a bit tricky is to supplement the B12 adequately without causing mood swings due to the COMT + + status. You will want to use hydroxy B12 rather than methyl B12 in an effort to reduce behavioral problems. The balance that has worked well in similar situations in the past is to start with one hydroxy B12 daily. Over the course of a week or two increase the hydroxy B12 first to 2 per day, and then to 3 per day. If you are seeing mood swings, then decrease the hydroxy B12 and move up more slowly in dosage. Literature suggests that oral B12 is as effective as injected B12; however as an alternative you can consider B12 injections. If you decide to use B12 injections it is preferable to use plain hydroxy B12 (no folinic or NAC). If you choose to use B12 injections it may be worth considering the addition of the chewable hydroxy B12 on the injections "off days". If you choose to use injections you can start with injections once a week and gradually increase to injections three times per week. This can be a very gradual process that is dictated by what he/she is able to tolerate; again using chewable B12 on the off days. If you decide to simply use the chewable hydroxy B12 this is an acceptable alternative. You may also want to add sublingual cyano B12 (once a day) to help to support his/her eyes.

As the level of B12 becomes more in balance following appropriate supplementation to address the methionine synthase mutation it will also help in balancing glutamate and gaba levels. In addition gaba can be added directly. Given the COMT and VDR status the use of plain gaba is suggested rather than ZEN, as the theanine in ZEN contains methyl groups.

There is a second pathway to the formation of methionine through the BHMT enzyme that will bypass this mutation. This pathway uses phosphatidyl serine and /or TMG as donors for the reaction. It is wise to consider adding PS and a small amount of TMG to help to drive this reaction. While DMG works well to support language, it may be best to wait to add any DMG until this pathway is supplemented properly, as the DMG may be inhibiting this BHMT reaction to methionine. Supplementation for this part of the pathway also uses a low dose of TMG, choline and plain methionine. The HHC general vitamin is acceptable as a source for TMG, choline and methionine as well as the other general nutrients contained in it (½-1 in the morning and another ½-1 in the afternoon). In addition, phosphatidyl serine should also be added to help to support the "back door" reaction from homocysteine to methionine via the BHMT enzyme. Phosphatidyl serine is available as plain PS gel caps as well as a chewable form with DMAE (Pedi-Active). DMAE contains methyl groups so the plain PS gel caps are the preferred form of this supplement rather than the chewable form given the COMT and VDR status. If even the use of plain PS seems to be a problem in terms of mood swings or depression then simply use the low doses of the HHC general vitamin. This will help to support the alternative pathway that will bypass the mutations in the MTR gene.

To summarize at this point, due to the COMT and VDR status appropriate methylation supplementation should include ¼ Folapro, ¼ Intrinsic B12, hydroxy B12, ¼ nucleotides, and ¼ dropper Methylation Support RNA, one to two of the HHC general vitamins, and a plain phosphatidyl serine gel cap. If mood swings occur then discontinue the use of phosphatidyl serine, also decrease the dose of hydroxy B12 and decrease the Folapro to 1/8 per day if needed. The biggest issue for him/her will be balancing the need for these methylation supplements, yet at the same time preventing mood swings due to dopamine excess. You will want to avoid the use of additional methyl donors which include curcumin, melatonin, FgF, theanine, ZEN, and MSM, SAMe, and methyl B12.

As the level of B12 becomes more in balance following appropriate methylation cycle supplementation it will also help in balancing glutamate and GABA levels. In addition plain GABA can be added directly. Plain GABA will be tolerated the best due to the COMT and VDR status. Where he/she is COMT + + or COMT + - VDR Bsm/Taq - - he/she will not be able to tolerate ZEN which contains theanine in addition to GABA. There are several other supplements that are very useful for balancing glutamate and GABA; these include taurine, pycnogenol and grape seed extract. These three are included in the general vitamin; however you may want to consider adding in additional amounts of pycnogenol, grape seed extract and taurine (except for no additional taurine for those with a CBS C699T+ mutation) as needed based on behavior especially as there are only very low doses of these in the general vitamin. GABA levels are related to language, as well as to anxiety levels, particularly anxiety in response to low blood sugar.

Lead inhibits a critical enzyme in the pathway for heme synthesis. A block in this pathway creates a build up of an intermediate that competes with GABA. Reduced GABA activity can cause auditory processing issues as well as language problems, and anxiety. In addition, inhibition of this pathway by lead can cause anemia, as well as the inability to make groups that are needed for B12 synthesis. A lack of these groups will exacerbate mutations in methionine synthase and methionine synthase reductase. This again points to the need for added B12 for individuals with mutations in this portion of the methylation cycle as well as the use of supplements to address lead toxicity in the body. The use of weekly baths in Beyond Clean, which contains EDTA should help to address lead toxicity in a very gentle manner that is suitable to most systems. It is also valuable to consider the use of ½ EDTA capsule per day or the use of EDTA chewing gum.

Once the methylation cycle is supplemented properly you may begin to see an increased level of detoxification. Generally there will be a one week "honeymoon" period followed by a regression in behaviors as the creatinine starts to climb. In order to monitor this and to understand changes in behavior that may occur as a result of this detoxification, it is a good idea to take spot urine samples and run urine toxic metal tests. It may seem like a supplement is non ideal for an individual. However, it is difficult to tell the difference between a negative reaction to a supplement and the behavioral impact of detoxification or a mood swing due to dopamine fluxes as the methylation pathway is supplemented properly; that is why use of regular urine toxic metal tests is so critical. The urine samples will help to separate the effects of methylation support on detoxification from supplements that do not agree with an individual.

- COMT + - VDR Bsm/Taq - -
- MTRR + or + +

There is a mutation in the methionine synthase reductase gene (MS_MTRR or MSR). The function of MSR is to regenerate B12 for the MS to utilize. What this means in practical terms is that he/she may be deficient in methyl B12. The supplementation of B12 is therefore very important for him/her. What will be a bit tricky is to supplement the B12 adequately without causing mood swings due to the COMT + + status. You will want to use hydroxy B12 rather than methyl B12 in an effort to reduce behavioral problems. The balance that has worked well in similar situations in the past is to start with one hydroxy B12 daily. Over the course of a week or two increase the hydroxy B12 first to 2 per day, and then to 3 per day. If you are seeing mood swings, then decrease the hydroxy B12 and move up more slowly in dosage. Literature suggests that oral B12 is as effective as injected B12; however as an alternative you can consider B12 injections. If you decide to use B12 injections it is preferable to use plain hydroxy B12 (no folinic or NAC). If you choose to use B12 injections it may be worth considering the addition of the chewable hydroxy B12 on the injections "off days". If you choose to use injections you can start with injections once a week and gradually increase to injections three times per week. This can be a very gradual process that is dictated by what he/she is able to tolerate; again using chewable B12 on the off days. If you decide to simply use the chewable hydroxy B12 this is an acceptable alternative. You may also want to add sublingual cyano B12 (once a day) to help to support his/her eyes.

As the level of B12 becomes more in balance following appropriate supplementation to address the methionine synthase reductase mutation it will also help in balancing

glutamate and gaba levels. In addition gaba can be added directly. Given the COMT and VDR status the use of plain gaba is suggested rather than ZEN, as the theanine in ZEN contains methyl groups.

There is a second pathway to the formation of methionine through the BHMT enzyme that will bypass this mutation. This pathway uses phosphatidyl serine and /or TMG as donors for the reaction. It is wise to consider adding PS and a small amount of TMG to help to drive this reaction. While DMG works well to support language, it may be best to wait to add any DMG until this pathway is supplemented properly, as the DMG may be inhibiting this BHMT reaction to methionine. Supplementation for this part of the pathway also uses a low dose of TMG, choline and plain methionine. The HHC general vitamin is acceptable as a source for TMG, choline and methionine as well as the other general nutrients contained in it (½-1 in the morning and another ½-1 in the afternoon). In addition, phosphatidyl serine should also be added to help to support the "back door" reaction from homocysteine to methionine via the BHMT enzyme. Phosphatidyl serine is available as plain PS gel caps as well as a chewable form with DMAE (Pedi-Active). DMAE contains methyl groups so the plain PS gel caps are the preferred form of this supplement rather than the chewable form given the COMT and VDR status. If even the use of plain PS seems to be a problem in terms of mood swings or depression then simply use the low doses of the HHC general vitamin. This will help to support the alternative pathway that will bypass the mutation in the MS_MTRR gene.

To summarize at this point, due to the COMT and VDR status appropriate methylation supplementation should include ¼ Folapro, ¼ Intrinsic B12, hydroxy B12, ¼ nucleotides, and ¼ dropper Methylation Support RNA, one to two of the HHC general vitamins, and a plain phosphatidyl

serine gel cap. If mood swings occur then discontinue the use of phosphatidyl serine, also decrease the dose of hydroxy B12 and decrease the Folapro to 1/8 per day if needed. The biggest issue for him/her will be balancing the need for these methylation supplements, yet at the same time preventing mood swings due to dopamine excess. You will want to avoid the use of additional methyl donors which include curcumin, melatonin, FgF, theanine, ZEN, and MSM, SAMe, and methyl B12.

As the level of B12 becomes more in balance following appropriate methylation cycle supplementation it will also help in balancing glutamate and GABA levels. In addition plain GABA can be added directly. Plain GABA will be tolerated the best due to the COMT and VDR status. Where he/she is COMT + + or COMT + - VDR Bsm/Taq - - he/she will not be able to tolerate ZEN which contains theanine in addition to GABA. There are several other supplements that are very useful for balancing glutamate and GABA; these include taurine, pycnogenol and grape seed extract. These three are included in the general vitamin; however you may want to consider adding in additional amounts of pycnogenol, grape seed extract and taurine (except for no additional taurine for those with a CBS C699T+ mutation) as needed based on behavior especially as there are only very low doses of these in the general vitamin. GABA levels are related to language, as well as to anxiety levels, particularly anxiety in response to low blood sugar.

Lead inhibits a critical enzyme in the pathway for heme synthesis. A block in this pathway creates a build up of an intermediate that competes with GABA. Reduced GABA activity can cause auditory processing issues as well as language problems, and anxiety. In addition, inhibition of this pathway by lead can cause anemia, as well as the inability to make groups that are needed for B12 synthesis. A lack of

these groups will exacerbate mutations in methionine synthase and methionine synthase reductase. This again points to the need for added B12 for individuals with mutations in this portion of the methylation cycle as well as the use of supplements to address lead toxicity in the body. The use of weekly baths in Beyond Clean, which contains EDTA should help to address lead toxicity in a very gentle manner that is suitable to most systems. It is also valuable to consider the use of ½ EDTA capsule per day or the use of EDTA chewing gum.

Once the methylation cycle is supplemented properly you may begin to see an increased level of detoxification. Generally there will be a one week "honeymoon" period followed by a regression in behaviors as the creatinine starts to climb. In order to monitor this and to understand changes in behavior that may occur as a result of this detoxification, it is a good idea to take spot urine samples and run urine toxic metal tests. It may seem like a supplement is non ideal for an individual. However, it is difficult to tell the difference between a negative reaction to a supplement and the behavioral impact of detoxification or a mood swing due to dopamine fluxes as the methylation pathway is supplemented properly; that is why use of regular urine toxic metal tests is so critical. The urine samples will help to separate the effects of methylation support on detoxification from supplements that do not agree with an individual.

- COMT + - VDR Bsm/Taq - -
- MTR + or + +
- MTRR + or + +

There is a mutation in the methionine synthase reductase gene (MS_MTRR or MSR), as well as a mutation in the methionine synthase gene (MS or MTR). The function of MSR is to regenerate B12 for the MS to utilize. The methionine synthase mutation is an up regulation mutation that enhances the activity of the enzyme. This should cause the enzyme to use up added B12 at an even faster rate than normal. What this means in practical terms is that he/she may be severely deficient in methyl B12. What will be a bit tricky is to supplement the B12 adequately without causing mood swings due to the COMT + + status. You will want to use hydroxy B12 rather than methyl B12 in an effort to reduce behavioral problems. The balance that has worked well in similar situations in the past is to start with one hydroxy B12 daily. Over the course of a week or two increase the hydroxy B12 first to 2 per day, and then to 3 per day. If you are seeing mood swings, then decrease the hydroxy B12 and move up more slowly in dosage. Literature suggests that oral B12 is as effective as injected B12; however as an alternative you can consider B12 injections. If you decide to use B12 injections it is preferable to use plain hydroxy B12 (no folinic or NAC). If you choose to use B12 injections it may be worth considering the addition of the chewable hydroxy B12 on the injections "off days". If you choose to use injections you can start with injections once a week and gradually increase to injections three times per week. This can be a very gradual process that is dictated by what he/she is able to tolerate; again using chewable B12 on the off days. If you decide to simply use the chewable hydroxy B12 this is an acceptable alternative. You may also want to add sublingual cyano B12 (once a day) to help to support his/her eyes.

As the level of B12 becomes more in balance following appropriate supplementation to address the methionine synthase reductase mutation it will also help in balancing glutamate and gaba levels. In addition gaba can be added directly. Given the COMT and VDR status the use of plain gaba is suggested rather than ZEN, as the theanine in ZEN contains methyl groups.

There is a second pathway to the formation of methionine through the BHMT enzyme that will bypass this mutation. This pathway uses phosphatidyl serine and /or TMG as donors for the reaction. It is wise to consider adding PS and a small amount of TMG to help to drive this reaction. While DMG works well to support language, it may be best to wait to add any DMG until this pathway is supplemented properly, as the DMG may be inhibiting this BHMT reaction to methionine. Supplementation for this part of the pathway also uses a low dose of TMG, choline and plain methionine. The HHC general vitamin is acceptable as a source for TMG, choline and methionine as well as the other general nutrients contained in it (½-1 in the morning and another ½-1 in the afternoon). In addition, phosphatidyl serine should also be added to help to support the "back door" reaction from homocysteine to methionine via the BHMT enzyme. Phosphatidyl serine is available as plain PS gel caps as well as a chewable form with DMAE (Pedi-Active). DMAE contains methyl groups so the plain PS gel caps are the preferred form of this supplement rather than the chewable form given the COMT and VDR status. If even the use of plain PS seems to be a problem in terms of mood swings or depression then simply use the low doses of the HHC general vitamin. This will help to support the alternative pathway that will bypass the mutations in the MS_MTRR as well as the MTR genes.

To summarize at this point, due to the COMT and VDR status appropriate methylation supplementation should include ¼ Folapro, ¼ Intrinsic B12, hydroxy B12, ¼ nucleotides, and ¼ dropper Methylation Support RNA, one to two of the HHC general vitamins, and a plain phosphatidyl serine gel cap. If mood swings occur then discontinue the use of phosphatidyl serine, also decrease the dose of hydroxy B12 and decrease the Folapro to 1/8 per day if needed. The biggest issue for him/her will be balancing the need for these methylation supplements, yet at the same time preventing mood swings due to dopamine excess. You will want to avoid the use of additional methyl donors which include curcumin, melatonin, FgF, theanine, ZEN, and MSM, SAMe, and methyl B12.

As the level of B12 becomes more in balance following appropriate methylation cycle supplementation it will also help in balancing glutamate and GABA levels. In addition plain GABA can be added directly. Plain GABA will be tolerated the best due to the COMT and VDR status. Where he/she is COMT + + or COMT + - VDR Bsm/Taq - - he/she will not be able to tolerate ZEN which contains theanine in addition to GABA. There are several other supplements that are very useful for balancing glutamate and GABA; these include taurine, pycnogenol and grape seed extract. These three are included in the general vitamin; however you may want to consider adding in additional amounts of pycnogenol, grape seed extract and taurine (except for no additional taurine for those with a CBS C699T+ mutation) as needed based on behavior especially as there are only very low doses of these in the general vitamin. GABA levels are related to language, as well as to anxiety levels, particularly anxiety in response to low blood sugar.

Lead inhibits a critical enzyme in the pathway for heme synthesis. A block in this pathway creates a build up of an intermediate that competes with GABA. Reduced GABA activity can cause auditory processing issues as well as language problems, and anxiety. In addition, inhibition of this pathway by lead can cause anemia, as well as the inability to make groups that are needed for B12 synthesis. A lack of these groups will exacerbate mutations in methionine synthase and methionine synthase reductase. This again points to the need for added B12 for individuals with mutations in this portion of the methylation cycle as well as the use of supplements to address lead toxicity in the body. The use of weekly baths in Beyond Clean, which contains EDTA should help to address lead toxicity in a very gentle manner that is suitable to most systems. It is also valuable to consider the use of ½ EDTA capsule per day or the use of EDTA chewing gum.

Once the methylation cycle is supplemented properly you may begin to see an increased level of detoxification. Generally there will be a one week "honeymoon" period followed by a regression in behaviors as the creatinine starts to climb. In order to monitor this and to understand changes in behavior that may occur as a result of this detoxification, it is a good idea to take spot urine samples and run urine toxic metal tests. It may seem like a supplement is non ideal for an individual. However, it is difficult to tell the difference between a negative reaction to a supplement and the behavioral impact of detoxification or a mood swing due to dopamine fluxes as the methylation pathway is supplemented properly; that is why use of regular urine toxic metal tests is so critical. The urine samples will help to separate the effects of methylation support on detoxification from supplements that do not agree with an individual.

COMT + - VDR Bsm/Taq + -

- COMT + -   VDR Bsm/Taq + -

The nutrigenomics report for this individual shows a single mutation in the COMT gene. This means that he/she is COMT+ - so that they should be able to tolerate more methyl donors than individuals who are COMT + +, however it will still be important to watch the total number of methyl donors that are used in supplements as he/she is also VDR Bsm/Taq + -. What this means in practical terms is that because he/she is COMT + - and VDR Bsm/Taq + - , he/she will behave more like a COMT + + individual in terms of their responses to most methyl donors. This will mean that supporting dopamine levels may be less of an issue as we look at the overall supplement plan. However, the COMT + - status, as compared to a COMT + + indicates that he/she will still be able to break down dopamine more rapidly than a COMT + + individual and as such will still be depleting methyl groups from their methylation cycle in the process. What this means in practical terms is that because he/she is COMT + - and VDR Bsm/Taq + - you will be able to use a few more methyl donors in key places in his/her supplement program. However, please use caution in the use of methyl donors and pay careful attention to the total amount of methyl donors in the supplement plan. Too many methyl donors may cause he/she to have mood swings. Pay careful attention to lithium and iodine levels during any detoxification of heavy metals, as excretion of mercury can affect the levels of lithium and iodine. These essential minerals appear to play an important role in helping to balance mood swings that can occur as a result of dopamine fluxes. These dopamine fluxes are more of an issue in individuals who are COMT + -/VDR Bsm and Taq + -, than in those who are COMT - - and VDR / Bsm and Taq + +.

It is also important to pay attention to foods containing a high level of tyrosine that may increase dopamine levels. Tyrosine and tryptophan will compete with each other for transport into the cell. Tryptophan helps to support serotonin levels and tyrosine helps to support dopamine levels. Therefore it is wise to consider the list of high tryptophan and high dopamine foods and try to concentrate on more of the high tryptophan foods and to limit the intake of the high tyrosine foods in an effort to support serotonin levels and to prevent mood swings due to dopamine overload.

- COMT + - VDR Bsm/Taq + -
- MTRR + or + +

There is also a mutation in the methionine synthase reductase gene (MS_MTRR or MSR). The function of MSR is to regenerate B12 for the methionine synthase to utilize. What this means in practical terms is that he/she may be deficient in methyl B12. Supplementation can start with one chewable methyl B12 (5mg) daily. This can gradually be increased to two to three methyl B12 per day if he/she will tolerate it. If mood swings occur, then decrease the dose of methyl B12 back down to a more comfortable level. Literature suggests that oral B12 is as effective as injected B12; however as an alternative you can consider B12 injections. If you decide to use B12 injections it is preferable to use plain methyl B12 (no folinic or NAC). If you choose to use B12 injections it may be worth considering the addition of the chewable methyl B12 on the injections "off days". If you choose to use injections you can start with injections once a week and gradually increase to injections three times per week. This can be a very gradual process that is dictated by what he/she is able to tolerate; again using chewable B12 on the off days. If you decide to simply use the chewable methyl B12 this is an acceptable alternative. Where he/she is COMT + - and VDR Bsm/Taq + - he/she should be able to tolerate supplementation with methyl B12. However, if you are seeing mood swings, then it will be necessary to strike a balance between the use of methyl B12 and hydroxy B12. The hydroxy form of B12 will help to support the B12 imbalances without adding methyl groups. The hydroxy B12 is also available as a chewable tablet, as well as in an injectable form. Depending on the individual you may find that more hydroxy relative to methyl B12 is better tolerated. You may also want to add sublingual cyano B12 (once a day) to help to support his/her eyes.

There is a second pathway to the formation of methionine through the BHMT enzyme that will bypass this mutation in the methionine synthase reductase gene. This pathway uses phosphatidyl serine and /or TMG as donors for the reaction. It is wise to consider adding PS and a small amount of TMG to help to drive this reaction. While DMG works well to support language, it may be best to wait to add any DMG until this pathway is supplemented properly, as the DMG may be inhibiting this BHMT reaction to methionine. Supplementation for this part of the pathway also uses a low dose of TMG, choline and plain methionine. The HHC general vitamin is acceptable as a source for TMG, choline and methionine as well as the other general nutrients contained in it (½-1 in the morning and another ½-1 in the afternoon). In addition, phosphatidyl serine should also be added to help to support the "back door" reaction from homocysteine to methionine via the BHMT enzyme. Phosphatidyl serine is available as plain PS gel caps as well as a chewable form with DMAE (Pedi-Active). DMAE contains methyl groups so this is an ideal form for individuals who need extra methyl groups based on their COMT and VDR test results. Plain phosphatidyl serine is often available as a gelcap and this is a preferred form. Therefore if he/she will tolerate it, you should consider the use of one phosphatidyl serine gelcap as well as one of the chewable Pedi-Active PS with DMAE daily. This will help to support the alternative pathway that will bypass the mutation in the MTR gene.

Again, as with the methyl B12, if you find that this is more methyl groups than he/she can tolerate without causing mood swings, then eliminate the use of the Pedi-Active containing the DMAE.

To summarize at this point, due to the COMT + - status appropriate methylation supplementation would include: ¼ Folapro, ¼ Intrinsic B12, methyl B12, ¼ nucleotides, SAMe

(1/2 to one per day), ¼ dropper methylation support RNA, one plain phosphatidyl serine gel cap, one Pedi-Active chewable phosphatidyl serine with DMAE, and one to two of the HHC neurological health general vitamins daily. SAMe is a critical intermediate in numerous reactions in the body. SAMe is a sulfur containing compound that is a critical intermediate in the methylation methionine/folate cycle and also serves as a methyl donor in the body. If this is more methylation than he/she is able to handle, and he/she begins to exhibit mood swings, then you can adjust the balance between the use of methyl and hydroxy B12 to favor more hydroxy B12, and also decrease the dose of SAMe or eliminate it entirely. Conversely, in the future if he/she is tolerating methyl donors well, you can consider the use of other methyl donors. You may want to consider the use of curcumin, melatonin, FgF, theanine, ZEN, and MSM (not for those with CBS C699T + status) in addition to the specific methyl donors already listed (SAMe, methyl B12).

As the level of B12 becomes more in balance following appropriate supplementation to address the methylation cycle mutation it will also help in balancing glutamate and GABA levels. In addition GABA can be added directly. Plain GABA will be tolerated due to the COMT and VDR status. Where he/she is COMT + - he/she should also be able to tolerate, and benefit from low doses of ZEN which contains theanine in addition to GABA, as theanine has methyl groups. There are several other supplements that are very useful for balancing glutamate and GABA; these include taurine, pycnogenol and grape seed extract. These three are included in the general vitamin; however you may want to consider adding in additional amounts of pycnogenol, grape seed extract and taurine (except for no additional taurine for those with a CBS C699T+ mutation) as needed based on behavior especially as there are only very low doses of these in the general vitamin.

GABA levels are related to language, as well as to anxiety levels, particularly anxiety in response to low blood sugar.

Lead inhibits a critical enzyme in the pathway for heme synthesis. A block in this pathway creates a build up of an intermediate that competes with GABA. Reduced GABA activity can cause auditory processing issues as well as language problems, and anxiety. In addition, inhibition of this pathway by lead can cause anemia, as well as the inability to make groups that are needed for B12 synthesis. A lack of these groups will exacerbate mutations in methionine synthase and methionine synthase reductase. This again points to the need for added B12 for individuals with mutations in this portion of the methylation cycle as well as the use of supplements to address lead toxicity in the body. The use of weekly baths in Beyond Clean, which contains EDTA should help to address lead toxicity in a very gentle manner that is suitable to most systems. It is also valuable to consider the use of ½ EDTA capsule per day or the use of EDTA chewing gum.

Once the methylation cycle is supplemented properly you may begin to see an increased level of detoxification. Generally there will be a one week "honeymoon" period followed by a regression in behaviors as the creatinine starts to climb. In order to monitor this and to understand changes in behavior that may occur as a result of this detoxification, it is a good idea to take spot urine samples and run urine toxic metal tests. It may seem like a supplement is non ideal for an individual. However, it is difficult to tell the difference between a negative reaction to a supplement and the behavioral impact of detoxification or a mood swing due to dopamine fluxes as the methylation pathway is supplemented properly; that is why use of regular urine toxic metal tests is so critical. The urine samples will help to separate the effects of methylation support on detoxification from supplements that do not agree with an individual.

- COMT + - VDR Bsm/Taq + -
- MTR + or + +

There is a single mutation in the methionine synthase gene (MS or MTR). The methionine synthase mutation is an up regulation mutation that enhances the activity of the enzyme. This should cause the enzyme to use up added methyl B12 at an even faster rate than normal. What this means in practical terms is that he/she may be deficient in methyl B12. Supplementation can start with one chewable methyl B12 (5mg) daily. This can gradually be increased to two to three methyl B12 per day if he/she will tolerate it. If mood swings occur, then decrease the dose of methyl B12 back down to a more comfortable level. Literature suggests that oral B12 is as effective as injected B12; however as an alternative you can consider B12 injections. If you decide to use B12 injections it is preferable to use plain methyl B12 (no folinic or NAC). If you choose to use B12 injections it may be worth considering the addition of the chewable methyl B12 on the injections "off days". If you choose to use injections you can start with injections once a week and gradually increase to injections three times per week. This can be a very gradual process that is dictated by what he/she is able to tolerate; again using chewable B12 on the off days. If you decide to simply use the chewable methyl B12 this is an acceptable alternative. Where he/she is COMT + - and VDR Bsm/Taq + - he/she should be able to tolerate supplementation with methyl B12. However, if you are seeing mood swings, then it will be necessary to strike a balance between the use of methyl B12 and hydroxy B12. The hydroxy form of B12 will help to support the B12 imbalances without adding methyl groups. The hydroxy B12 is also available as a chewable tablet, as well as in an injectable form. Depending on the individual you may find that more hydroxy relative to methyl B12 is better tolerated. You may also want to add sublingual cyano B12 (once a day) to help to support his/her eyes.

There is a second pathway to the formation of methionine through the BHMT enzyme that will bypass this mutation in the methionine synthase gene. This pathway uses phosphatidyl serine and /or TMG as donors for the reaction. It is wise to consider adding PS and a small amount of TMG to help to drive this reaction. While DMG works well to support language, it may be best to wait to add any DMG until this pathway is supplemented properly, as the DMG may be inhibiting this BHMT reaction to methionine. Supplementation for this part of the pathway also uses a low dose of TMG, choline and plain methionine. The HHC general vitamin is acceptable as a source for TMG, choline and methionine as well as the other general nutrients contained in it (½-1 in the morning and another ½-1 in the afternoon). In addition, phosphatidyl serine should also be added to help to support the "back door" reaction from homocysteine to methionine via the BHMT enzyme. Phosphatidyl serine is available as plain PS gel caps as well as a chewable form with DMAE (Pedi-Active). DMAE contains methyl groups so this is an ideal form for individuals who need extra methyl groups based on their COMT and VDR test results. Plain phosphatidyl serine is often available as a gelcap and this is a preferred form. Therefore if he/she will tolerate it, you should consider the use of one phosphatidyl serine gelcap as well as one of the chewable Pedi-Active PS with DMAE daily. This will help to support the alternative pathway that will bypass the mutation in the MTR gene.

Again, as with the methyl B12, if you find that this is more methyl groups than he/she can tolerate without causing mood swings, then eliminate the use of the Pedi-Active containing the DMAE.

To summarize at this point, due to the COMT + - status appropriate methylation supplementation would include: ¼ Folapro, ¼ Intrinsic B12, methyl B12, ¼ nucleotides, SAMe (1/2 to one per day), ¼ dropper methylation support RNA, one plain phosphatidyl serine gel cap, one Pedi-Active chewable phosphatidyl serine with DMAE, and one to two of the HHC neurological health general vitamins daily. SAMe is a critical intermediate in numerous reactions in the body. SAMe is a sulfur containing compound that is a critical intermediate in the methylation methionine/folate cycle and also serves as a methyl donor in the body. If this is more methylation than he/she is able to handle, and he/she begins to exhibit mood swings, then you can adjust the balance between the use of methyl and hydroxy B12 to favor more hydroxy B12, and also decrease the dose of SAMe or eliminate it entirely. Conversely, in the future if he/she is tolerating methyl donors well, you can consider the use of other methyl donors. You may want to consider the use of curcumin, melatonin, FgF, theanine, ZEN, and MSM (not for those with CBS C699T + status) in addition to the specific methyl donors already listed (SAMe, methyl B12).

As the level of B12 becomes more in balance following appropriate supplementation to address the methylation cycle mutation it will also help in balancing glutamate and GABA levels. In addition GABA can be added directly. Plain GABA will be tolerated due to the COMT and VDR status. Where he/she is COMT + - he/she should also be able to tolerate, and benefit from low doses of ZEN which contains theanine in addition to GABA, as theanine has methyl groups. There are several other supplements that are very useful for balancing glutamate and GABA; these include taurine, pycnogenol and grape seed extract. These three are included in the general vitamin; however you may want to consider adding in additional amounts of pycnogenol, grape seed extract and taurine (except for _no_ additional taurine for those with a CBS

C699T+ mutation) as needed based on behavior especially as there are only very low doses of these in the general vitamin. GABA levels are related to language, as well as to anxiety levels, particularly anxiety in response to low blood sugar.

Lead inhibits a critical enzyme in the pathway for heme synthesis. A block in this pathway creates a build up of an intermediate that competes with GABA. Reduced GABA activity can cause auditory processing issues as well as language problems, and anxiety. In addition, inhibition of this pathway by lead can cause anemia, as well as the inability to make groups that are needed for B12 synthesis. A lack of these groups will exacerbate mutations in methionine synthase and methionine synthase reductase. This again points to the need for added B12 for individuals with mutations in this portion of the methylation cycle as well as the use of supplements to address lead toxicity in the body. The use of weekly baths in Beyond Clean, which contains EDTA should help to address lead toxicity in a very gentle manner that is suitable to most systems. It is also valuable to consider the use of ½ EDTA capsule per day or the use of EDTA chewing gum.

Once the methylation cycle is supplemented properly you may begin to see an increased level of detoxification. Generally there will be a one week "honeymoon" period followed by a regression in behaviors as the creatinine starts to climb. In order to monitor this and to understand changes in behavior that may occur as a result of this detoxification, it is a good idea to take spot urine samples and run urine toxic metal tests. It may seem like a supplement is non ideal for an individual. However, it is difficult to tell the difference between a negative reaction to a supplement and the behavioral impact of detoxification or a mood swing due to dopamine fluxes as the methylation pathway is supplemented properly; that is why use of regular urine toxic metal tests is so critical. The urine samples will help to separate the effects of methylation support on detoxification from supplements that do not agree with an individual.

To summarize at this point, due to the COMT + - status appropriate methylation supplementation would include: ¼ Folapro, ¼ Intrinsic B12, methyl B12, ¼ nucleotides, SAMe (1/2 to one per day), ¼ dropper methylation support RNA, one plain phosphatidyl serine gel cap, one Pedi-Active chewable phosphatidyl serine with DMAE, and one to two of the HHC neurological health general vitamins daily. SAMe is a critical intermediate in numerous reactions in the body. SAMe is a sulfur containing compound that is a critical intermediate in the methylation methionine/folate cycle and also serves as a methyl donor in the body. If this is more methylation than he/she is able to handle, and he/she begins to exhibit mood swings, then you can adjust the balance between the use of methyl and hydroxy B12 to favor more hydroxy B12, and also decrease the dose of SAMe or eliminate it entirely. Conversely, in the future if he/she is tolerating methyl donors well, you can consider the use of other methyl donors. You may want to consider the use of curcumin, melatonin, FgF, theanine, ZEN, and MSM (not for those with CBS C699T + status) in addition to the specific methyl donors already listed (SAMe, methyl B12).

As the level of B12 becomes more in balance following appropriate supplementation to address the methylation cycle mutation it will also help in balancing glutamate and GABA levels. In addition GABA can be added directly. Plain GABA will be tolerated due to the COMT and VDR status. Where he/she is COMT + - he/she should also be able to tolerate, and benefit from low doses of ZEN which contains theanine in addition to GABA, as theanine has methyl groups. There are several other supplements that are very useful for balancing glutamate and GABA; these include taurine, pycnogenol and grape seed extract. These three are included in the general vitamin; however you may want to consider adding in additional amounts of pycnogenol, grape seed extract and taurine (except for no additional taurine for those with a CBS C699T+ mutation) as needed based on behavior especially as there are only very low doses of these in the general vitamin. GABA levels are related to language, as well as to anxiety levels, particularly anxiety in response to low blood sugar.

Lead inhibits a critical enzyme in the pathway for heme synthesis. A block in this pathway creates a build up of an intermediate that competes with GABA. Reduced GABA activity can cause auditory processing issues as well as language problems, and anxiety. In addition, inhibition of this pathway by lead can cause anemia, as well as the inability to make groups that are needed for B12 synthesis. A lack of these groups will exacerbate mutations in methionine synthase and methionine synthase reductase. This again points to the need for added B12 for individuals with mutations in this portion of the methylation cycle as well as the use of supplements to address lead toxicity in the body. The use of weekly baths in Beyond Clean, which contains EDTA should help to address lead toxicity in a very gentle manner that is suitable to most systems. It is also valuable to consider the use of ½ EDTA capsule per day or the use of EDTA chewing gum.

Once the methylation cycle is supplemented properly you may begin to see an increased level of detoxification. Generally there will be a one week "honeymoon" period followed by a regression in behaviors as the creatinine starts to climb. In order to monitor this and to understand changes in behavior that may occur as a result of this detoxification, it is a good idea to take spot urine samples and run urine toxic metal tests. It may seem like a supplement is non ideal for an individual. However, it is difficult to tell the difference between a negative reaction to a supplement and the behavioral impact of detoxification or a mood swing due to dopamine fluxes as the methylation pathway is supplemented properly; that is why use of regular urine toxic metal tests is so critical. The urine samples will help to separate the effects of methylation support on detoxification from supplements that do not agree with an individual.

- COMT + - VDR Bsm/Taq + -
- MTR + or + +
- MTRR + or + +

There is also a mutation in the methionine synthase reductase gene (MS_MTRR or MSR), as well as a mutation in the methionine synthase gene (MS or MTR). The function of MSR is to regenerate B12 for the MS to utilize. The methionine synthase mutation is an up regulation mutation that enhances the activity of the enzyme. This should cause the enzyme to use up added B12 at an even faster rate than normal. What this means in practical terms is that he/she may be severely deficient in methyl B12. Supplementation can start with one chewable methyl B12 (5mg) daily. This can gradually be increased to two to three methyl B12 per day if he/she will tolerate it. If mood swings occur, then decrease the dose of methyl B12 back down to a more comfortable level. Literature suggests that oral B12 is as effective as injected B12; however as an alternative you can consider B12 injections. If you decide to use B12 injections it is preferable to use plain methyl B12 (no folinic or NAC). If you choose to use B12 injections it may be worth considering the addition of the chewable methyl B12 on the injections "off days". If you choose to use injections you can start with injections once a week and gradually increase to injections three times per week. This can be a very gradual process that is dictated by what he/she is able to tolerate; again using chewable B12 on the off days. If you decide to simply use the chewable methyl B12 this is an acceptable alternative. Where he/she is COMT + - and VDR Bsm/Taq + - he/she should be able to tolerate supplementation with methyl B12. However, if you are seeing mood swings, then it will be necessary to strike a balance between the use of methyl B12 and hydroxy B12. The hydroxy form of B12 will help to support the B12 imbalances without adding methyl groups. The hydroxy B12 is also available as a chewable tablet, as well as in an injectable form. Depending on the individual you may find that more hydroxy relative to methyl B12 is better tolerated. You may also want to add sublingual cyano B12 (once a day) to help to support his/her eyes.

There is a second pathway to the formation of methionine through the BHMT enzyme that will bypass both these mutations in the methionine synthase reductase gene and the methionine synthase genes. This pathway uses phosphatidyl serine and /or TMG as donors for the reaction. It is wise to consider adding PS and a small amount of TMG to help to drive this reaction. While DMG works well to support language, it may be best to wait to add any DMG until this pathway is supplemented properly, as the DMG may be inhibiting this BHMT reaction to methionine. Supplementation for this part of the pathway also uses a low dose of TMG, choline and plain methionine. The HHC general vitamin is acceptable as a source for TMG, choline and methionine as well as the other general nutrients contained in it (½-1 in the morning and another ½-1 in the afternoon). In addition, phosphatidyl serine should also be added to help to support the "back door" reaction from homocysteine to methionine via the BHMT enzyme. Phosphatidyl serine is available as plain PS gel caps as well as a chewable form with DMAE (Pedi-Active). DMAE contains methyl groups so this is an ideal form for individuals who need extra methyl groups based on their COMT and VDR test results. Plain phosphatidyl serine is often available as a gelcap and this is a preferred form. Therefore if he/she will tolerate it, you should consider the use of one phosphatidyl serine gelcap as well as one of the chewable Pedi-Active PS with DMAE daily. This will help to support the alternative pathway that will bypass the mutations in the MTR and MS_MTRR genes.

Again, as with the methyl B12, if you find that this is more methyl groups than he/she can tolerate without causing mood swings, then eliminate the use of the Pedi-Active containing the DMAE.

To summarize at this point, due to the COMT + - status appropriate methylation supplementation would include: ¼ Folapro, ¼ Intrinsic B12, methyl B12, ¼ nucleotides, SAMe (1/2 to one per day), ¼ dropper methylation support RNA, one plain phosphatidyl serine gel cap, one Pedi-Active chewable phosphatidyl serine with DMAE, and one to two of the HHC neurological health general vitamins daily. SAMe is a critical intermediate in numerous reactions in the body. SAMe is a sulfur containing compound that is a critical intermediate in the methylation methionine/folate cycle and also serves as a methyl donor in the body. If this is more methylation than he/she is able to handle, and he/she begins to exhibit mood swings, then you can adjust the balance between the use of methyl and hydroxy B12 to favor more hydroxy B12, and also decrease the dose of SAMe or eliminate it entirely. Conversely, in the future if he/she is tolerating methyl donors well, you can consider the use of other methyl donors. You may want to consider the use of curcumin, melatonin, FgF, theanine, ZEN, and MSM (not for those with CBS C699T + status) in addition to the specific methyl donors already listed (SAMe, methyl B12).

As the level of B12 becomes more in balance following appropriate supplementation to address the methylation cycle mutation it will also help in balancing glutamate and GABA levels. In addition GABA can be added directly. Plain GABA will be tolerated due to the COMT and VDR status. Where he/she is COMT + - he/she should also be able to tolerate, and benefit from low doses of ZEN which contains theanine in addition to GABA, as theanine has methyl groups. There are several other supplements that are very useful for balancing glutamate and GABA; these include taurine, pycnogenol and grape seed extract. These three are included in the general vitamin; however you may want to consider adding in additional amounts of pycnogenol, grape seed extract and taurine (except for no additional taurine for those with a CBS C699T+ mutation) as needed based on behavior especially as there are only very low doses of these in the general vitamin. GABA levels are related to language, as well as to anxiety levels, particularly anxiety in response to low blood sugar.

Lead inhibits a critical enzyme in the pathway for heme synthesis. A block in this pathway creates a build up of an intermediate that competes with GABA. Reduced GABA activity can cause auditory processing issues as well as language problems, and anxiety. In addition, inhibition of this pathway by lead can cause anemia, as well as the inability to make groups that are needed for B12 synthesis. A lack of these groups will exacerbate mutations in methionine synthase and methionine synthase reductase. This again points to the need for added B12 for individuals with mutations in this portion of the methylation cycle as well as the use of supplements to address lead toxicity in the body. The use of weekly baths in Beyond Clean, which contains EDTA should help to address lead toxicity in a very gentle manner that is suitable to most systems. It is also valuable to consider the use of ½ EDTA capsule per day or the use of EDTA chewing gum.

Once the methylation cycle is supplemented properly you may begin to see an increased level of detoxification. Generally there will be a one week "honeymoon" period followed by a regression in behaviors as the creatinine starts to climb. In order to monitor this and to understand changes in behavior that may occur as a result of this detoxification, it is a good idea to take spot urine samples and run urine toxic metal tests. It may seem like a supplement is non ideal for an individual. However, it is difficult to tell the difference between a negative reaction to a supplement and the behavioral impact of detoxification or a mood swing due to dopamine fluxes as the methylation pathway is supplemented properly; that is why use of regular urine toxic metal tests is so critical. The urine samples will help to separate the effects of methylation support on detoxification from supplements that do not agree with an individual.

COMT + - VDR Bsm/Taq + +

- COMT + - VDR Bsm/Taq + +

The nutrigenomics report for this individual shows a single mutation in the COMT gene. This means that he/she is COMT+ - so that he/she should be able to tolerate more methyl donors than individuals who are COMT + +, it will still be important to watch the total number of methyl donors that are used in supplements. The COMT + - status indicates that he/she will break down dopamine more rapidly than a COMT + + individual and as such will be depleting methyl groups from his/her methylation cycle in the process, although not to the extent that we see with COMT- - individuals. This individual is also VDR Bsm/Taq + +. What this means in practical terms is that because he/she is COMT + - and VDR Bsm/Taq + + he/she will behave like a COMT - - individual in terms of their responses to most methyl donors and may need added methyl donors for optimal dopamine and other methyl balance in the body. In addition, his/her toxic metal and viral burden may be higher than a individual who is COMT + + and VDR Bsm/Taq - -. As a result it may take a little longer to excrete all of the necessary metals and virus for optimal health.

It would make sense for this individual to eat a balance of high tryptophan foods and high tyrosine foods in an effort to support serotonin and dopamine levels. Tyrosine and tryptophan will compete with each other for transport into the cell. Tryptophan helps to support serotonin levels and tyrosine helps to support dopamine levels. Therefore if a balance of foods is used it will help to support healthy levels of both neurotransmitters. You can also consider the use of supplements to help to support healthy neurotransmitter levels. This would include using ¼ Mood S RNA once or twice per day and the use of St. John's Wort. This herb has some antiviral effects. In addition it is reported to help prevent the breakdown of serotonin. The use of small amounts of the

Mood D and the Mood Focus RNA may be helpful to support healthy dopamine levels. Due to the COMT + - status, the suggested use is only 1/8 dropper per day. In addition to the Mood Focus and Mood D RNA consider supplementing with quercetin. This will help to support healthy dopamine levels and will help to limit allergic reactions in the body. Consider starting with 1/2 quercetin per day. Ginkgo has been reported to help to increase dopamine uptake; again the suggested starting point is ½ ginkgo per day. There is also a natural source of dopamine that is available that is an extract from Mucuna Pruriens. You could consider a very small sprinkle of this product however large doses are not suggested. Where he/she is VDR Bsm/Taq + + and COMT + - a benefit should be derived from low doses of supplements to support healthy dopamine levels as described above. However, if there are mood swings as a result of the supplements to support dopamine levels then you will want to decrease the dopamine supplements to half their initial dose in order to prevent future mood swings.

- COMT + - VDR Bsm/Taq + +
- MTRR + or + +

There is also a mutation in the methionine synthase reductase gene (MS_MTRR or MSR). What this means in practical terms is that he/she may be deficient in methyl B12. The function of MSR is to regenerate B12 for the methionine synthase to utilize. Due to his/her COMT and VDR Bsm/Taq status he/she should need and will tolerate the addition of methyl containing supplements. Supplementation with methyl B12 should be beneficial for him/her. This will both help to support the MTR mutation as well as to add methyl groups to his/her system. Supplementation can start with one chewable methyl B12 (5mg) daily. This can gradually be increased to two to three methyl B12 per day if he/she will tolerate it. If mood swings occur, then decrease the dose of methyl B12 back down to a more comfortable level. Literature suggests that oral B12 is as effective as injected B12; however as an alternative you can consider B12 injections. If you decide to use B12 injections it is preferable to use plain methyl B12 (no folinic or NAC). If you choose to use B12 injections it may be worth considering the addition of the chewable methyl B12 on the injections "off days". If you choose to use injections you can start with injections once a week and gradually increase to injections three times per week. This can be a very gradual process that is dictated by what he/she is able to tolerate; again using chewable B12 on the off days. If you decide to simply use the chewable methyl B12 this is an acceptable alternative. You may also want to add sublingual cyano B12 (once a day) to help to support his/her eyes.

There is a second pathway to the formation of methionine through the BHMT enzyme that will bypass this mutation in the methionine synthase reductase gene. This pathway uses phosphatidyl serine and /or TMG as donors for the reaction. It

is wise to consider adding PS and a small amount of TMG to help to drive this reaction. While DMG works well to support language, it may be best to wait to add any DMG until this pathway is supplemented properly, as the DMG may be inhibiting this BHMT reaction to methionine. Supplementation for this part of the pathway also uses a low dose of TMG, choline and plain methionine. The HHC general vitamin is acceptable as a source for TMG, choline and methionine as well as the other general nutrients contained in it (½-1 in the morning and another ½-1 in the afternoon). In addition, phosphatidyl serine should also be added to help to support the "back door" reaction from homocysteine to methionine via the BHMT enzyme. Phosphatidyl serine is available as plain PS gel caps as well as a chewable form with DMAE (Pedi-Active). DMAE contains methyl groups so this is an ideal form for individuals who need extra methyl groups based on their COMT and VDR test results. Plain phosphatidyl serine is often available as a gelcap and this is a preferred form. Therefore if he/she will tolerate it, you should consider the use of one phosphatidyl serine gelcap as well as one of the chewable Pedi-Active PS with DMAE daily. This will help to support the alternative pathway that will bypass the mutation in the MTR gene.

Again, as with the methyl B12, if you find that this is more methyl groups than he/she can tolerate without causing mood swings, then eliminate the use of the Pedi-Active containing the DMAE.

To summarize at this point, due to the COMT + - status appropriate methylation supplementation would include: ¼ Folapro, ¼ Intrinsic B12, methyl B12, ¼ nucleotides, SAMe (1/2 to one per day), ¼ dropper methylation support RNA, one plain phosphatidyl serine gel cap, one Pedi-Active chewable phosphatidyl serine with DMAE, and one to two of the HHC neurological health general vitamins daily. SAMe is a critical intermediate in numerous reactions in the body. SAMe is a sulfur containing compound that is a critical intermediate in the methylation methionine/folate cycle and also serves as a methyl donor in the body. If this is more methylation than he/she is able to handle, and he/she begins to exhibit mood swings, then you can adjust the balance between the use of methyl and hydroxy B12 to favor more hydroxy B12, and also decrease the dose of SAMe or eliminate it entirely. Conversely, in the future if he/she is tolerating methyl donors well, you can consider the use of other methyl donors. You may want to consider the use of curcumin, melatonin, FgF, theanine, ZEN, and MSM (not for those with CBS C699T + status) in addition to the specific methyl donors already listed (SAMe, methyl B12).

As the level of B12 becomes more in balance following appropriate supplementation to address the methylation cycle mutation it will also help in balancing glutamate and GABA levels. In addition GABA can be added directly. Plain GABA will be tolerated due to the COMT and VDR status. Where he/she is COMT + - he/she should also be able to tolerate, and benefit from low doses of ZEN which contains theanine in addition to GABA, as theanine has methyl groups. There are several other supplements that are very useful for balancing glutamate and GABA; these include taurine, pycnogenol and grape seed extract. These three are included in the general vitamin; however you may want to consider adding in additional amounts of pycnogenol, grape seed extract and taurine (except for _no_ additional taurine for those with a CBS C699T+ mutation) as needed based on behavior especially as there are only very low doses of these in the general vitamin. GABA levels are related to language, as well as to anxiety levels, particularly anxiety in response to low blood sugar.

Lead inhibits a critical enzyme in the pathway for heme synthesis. A block in this pathway creates a build up of an

intermediate that competes with GABA. Reduced GABA activity can cause auditory processing issues as well as language problems, and anxiety. In addition, inhibition of this pathway by lead can cause anemia, as well as the inability to make groups that are needed for B12 synthesis. A lack of these groups will exacerbate mutations in methionine synthase and methionine synthase reductase. This again points to the need for added B12 for individuals with mutations in this portion of the methylation cycle as well as the use of supplements to address lead toxicity in the body. The use of weekly baths in Beyond Clean, which contains EDTA should help to address lead toxicity in a very gentle manner that is suitable to most systems. It is also valuable to consider the use of ½ EDTA capsule per day or the use of EDTA chewing gum.

Once the methylation cycle is supplemented properly you may begin to see an increased level of detoxification. Generally there will be a one week "honeymoon" period followed by a regression in behaviors as the creatinine starts to climb. In order to monitor this and to understand changes in behavior that may occur as a result of this detoxification, it is a good idea to take spot urine samples and run urine toxic metal tests. It may seem like a supplement is non ideal for an individual. However, it is difficult to tell the difference between a negative reaction to a supplement and the behavioral impact of detoxification or a mood swing due to dopamine fluxes as the methylation pathway is supplemented properly; that is why use of regular urine toxic metal tests is so critical. The urine samples will help to separate the effects of methylation support on detoxification from supplements that do not agree with an individual.

- COMT + - VDR Bsm/Taq + +
- MTR + or + +

There is a single mutation in the methionine synthase gene (MS or MTR). The methionine synthase mutation is an up regulation mutation that enhances the activity of the enzyme. This should cause the enzyme to use up added methyl B12 at an even faster rate than normal. What this means in practical terms is that he/she may be deficient in methyl B12. Due to his/her COMT and VDR Bsm/Taq status he/she should need and will tolerate the addition of methyl containing supplements. Supplementation with methyl B12 should be beneficial for him/her. This will both help to support the MTR mutation as well as to add methyl groups to his/her system. Supplementation can start with one chewable methyl B12 (5mg) daily. This can gradually be increased to two to three methyl B12 per day if he/she will tolerate it. If mood swings occur, then decrease the dose of methyl B12 back down to a more comfortable level. Literature suggests that oral B12 is as effective as injected B12; however as an alternative you can consider B12 injections. If you decide to use B12 injections it is preferable to use plain methyl B12 (no folinic or NAC). If you choose to use B12 injections it may be worth considering the addition of the chewable methyl B12 on the injections "off days". If you choose to use injections you can start with injections once a week and gradually increase to injections three times per week. This can be a very gradual process that is dictated by what he/she is able to tolerate; again using chewable B12 on the off days. If you decide to simply use the chewable methyl B12 this is an acceptable alternative. You may also want to add sublingual cyano B12 (once a day) to help to support his/her eyes.

There is a second pathway to the formation of methionine through the BHMT enzyme that will bypass this mutation in

the methionine synthase gene. This pathway uses phosphatidyl serine and /or TMG as donors for the reaction. It is wise to consider adding PS and a small amount of TMG to help to drive this reaction. While DMG works well to support language, it may be best to wait to add any DMG until this pathway is supplemented properly, as the DMG may be inhibiting this BHMT reaction to methionine. Supplementation for this part of the pathway also uses a low dose of TMG, choline and plain methionine. The HHC general vitamin is acceptable as a source for TMG, choline and methionine as well as the other general nutrients contained in it (½-1 in the morning and another ½-1 in the afternoon). In addition, phosphatidyl serine should also be added to help to support the "back door" reaction from homocysteine to methionine via the BHMT enzyme. Phosphatidyl serine is available as plain PS gel caps as well as a chewable form with DMAE (Pedi-Active). DMAE contains methyl groups so this is an ideal form for individuals who need extra methyl groups based on their COMT and VDR test results. Plain phosphatidyl serine is often available as a gelcap and this is a preferred form. Therefore if he/she will tolerate it, you should consider the use of one phosphatidyl serine gelcap as well as one of the chewable Pedi-Active PS with DMAE daily. This will help to support the alternative pathway that will bypass the mutation in the MTR gene.

Again, as with the methyl B12, if you find that this is more methyl groups than he/she can tolerate without causing mood swings, then eliminate the use of the Pedi-Active containing the DMAE.

To summarize at this point, due to the COMT + - status appropriate methylation supplementation would include: ¼ Folapro, ¼ Intrinsic B12, methyl B12, ¼ nucleotides, SAMe (1/2 to one per day), ¼ dropper methylation support RNA, one plain phosphatidyl serine gel cap, one Pedi-Active chewable phosphatidyl serine with DMAE, and one to two of the HHC neurological health general vitamins daily. SAMe is a critical intermediate in numerous reactions in the body. SAMe is a sulfur containing compound that is a critical intermediate in the methylation methionine/folate cycle and also serves as a methyl donor in the body. If this is more methylation than he/she is able to handle, and he/she begins to exhibit mood swings, then you can adjust the balance between the use of methyl and hydroxy B12 to favor more hydroxy B12, and also decrease the dose of SAMe or eliminate it entirely. Conversely, in the future if he/she is tolerating methyl donors well, you can consider the use of other methyl donors. You may want to consider the use of curcumin, melatonin, FgF, theanine, ZEN, and MSM (not for those with CBS C699T + status) in addition to the specific methyl donors already listed (SAMe, methyl B12).

As the level of B12 becomes more in balance following appropriate supplementation to address the methylation cycle mutation it will also help in balancing glutamate and GABA levels. In addition GABA can be added directly. Plain GABA will be tolerated due to the COMT and VDR status. Where he/she is COMT + - he/she should also be able to tolerate, and benefit from low doses of ZEN which contains theanine in addition to GABA, as theanine has methyl groups. There are several other supplements that are very useful for balancing glutamate and GABA; these include taurine, pycnogenol and grape seed extract. These three are included in the general vitamin; however you may want to consider adding in additional amounts of pycnogenol, grape seed extract and taurine (except for no additional taurine for those with a CBS C699T+ mutation) as needed based on behavior especially as there are only very low doses of these in the general vitamin. GABA levels are related to language, as well as to anxiety levels, particularly anxiety in response to low blood sugar.

Lead inhibits a critical enzyme in the pathway for heme synthesis. A block in this pathway creates a build up of an intermediate that competes with GABA. Reduced GABA activity can cause auditory processing issues as well as language problems, and anxiety. In addition, inhibition of this pathway by lead can cause anemia, as well as the inability to make groups that are needed for B12 synthesis. A lack of these groups will exacerbate mutations in methionine synthase and methionine synthase reductase. This again points to the need for added B12 for individuals with mutations in this portion of the methylation cycle as well as the use of supplements to address lead toxicity in the body. The use of weekly baths in Beyond Clean, which contains EDTA should help to address lead toxicity in a very gentle manner that is suitable to most systems. It is also valuable to consider the use of ½ EDTA capsule per day or the use of EDTA chewing gum.

Once the methylation cycle is supplemented properly you may begin to see an increased level of detoxification. Generally there will be a one week "honeymoon" period followed by a regression in behaviors as the creatinine starts to climb. In order to monitor this and to understand changes in behavior that may occur as a result of this detoxification, it is a good idea to take spot urine samples and run urine toxic metal tests. It may seem like a supplement is non ideal for an individual. However, it is difficult to tell the difference between a negative reaction to a supplement and the behavioral impact of detoxification or a mood swing due to dopamine fluxes as the methylation pathway is supplemented properly; that is why use of regular urine toxic metal tests is so critical. The urine samples will help to separate the effects of methylation support on detoxification from supplements that do not agree with an individual.

- COMT + - VDR Bsm/Taq + +
- MTR + or + +
- MTRR + or + +

There is also a mutation in the methionine synthase reductase gene (MS_MTRR or MSR), as well as a mutation in the methionine synthase gene (MS or MTR). The function of MSR is to regenerate B12 for the MS to utilize. The methionine synthase mutation is an up regulation mutation that enhances the activity of the enzyme. This should cause the enzyme to use up added B12 at an even faster rate than normal. What this means in practical terms is that he/she may be severely deficient in methyl B12. The supplementation of B12 is therefore very important for him/her. Due to his/her COMT and VDR Bsm/Taq status he/she should need and will tolerate the addition of methyl containing supplements. Supplementation with methyl B12 should be beneficial for him/her. This will both help to support the MTR mutation as well as to add methyl groups to his/her system.

Supplementation can start with one chewable methyl B12 (5mg) daily. This can gradually be increased to two to three methyl B12 per day if he/she will tolerate it. If mood swings occur, then decrease the dose of methyl B12 back down to a more comfortable level. Literature suggests that oral B12 is as effective as injected B12; however as an alternative you can consider B12 injections. If you decide to use B12 injections it is preferable to use plain methyl B12 (no folinic or NAC). If you choose to use B12 injections it may be worth considering the addition of the chewable methyl B12 on the injections "off days". If you choose to use injections you can start with injections once a week and gradually increase to injections three times per week. This can be a very gradual process that is dictated by what he/she is able to tolerate; again using chewable B12 on the off days. If you decide to simply use the chewable methyl B12 this is an acceptable alternative. You may also want to add sublingual cyano B12 (once a day) to help to support his/her eyes.

There is a second pathway to the formation of methionine through the BHMT enzyme that will bypass both of these mutations in the methionine synthase reductase and the methionine synthase genes. This pathway uses phosphatidyl serine and /or TMG as donors for the reaction. It is wise to consider adding PS and a small amount of TMG to help to drive this reaction. While DMG works well to support language, it may be best to wait to add any DMG until this pathway is supplemented properly, as the DMG may be inhibiting this BHMT reaction to methionine. Supplementation for this part of the pathway also uses a low dose of TMG, choline and plain methionine. The HHC general vitamin is acceptable as a source for TMG, choline and methionine as well as the other general nutrients contained in it (½-1 in the morning and another ½-1 in the afternoon). In addition, phosphatidyl serine should also be added to help to support the "back door" reaction from homocysteine to methionine via the BHMT enzyme. Phosphatidyl serine is available as plain PS gel caps as well as a chewable form with DMAE (Pedi-Active). DMAE contains methyl groups so this is an ideal form for individuals who need extra methyl groups based on their COMT and VDR test results. Plain phosphatidyl serine is often available as a gel cap and this is a preferred form. Therefore if he/she will tolerate it, you should consider the use of one phosphatidyl serine gel cap as well as one of the chewable Pedi-Active PS with DMAE daily. This will help to support the alternative pathway that will bypass the mutations in the MTR and MS_MTRR genes.

Again, as with the methyl B12, if you find that this is more methyl groups than he/she can tolerate without causing mood swings, then eliminate the use of the Pedi-Active containing the DMAE.

To summarize at this point, due to the COMT + - status appropriate methylation supplementation would include: ¼ Folapro, ¼ Intrinsic B12, methyl B12, ¼ nucleotides, SAMe (1/2 to one per day), ¼ dropper methylation support RNA, one plain phosphatidyl serine gel cap, one Pedi-Active chewable phosphatidyl serine with DMAE, and one to two of the HHC neurological health general vitamins daily. SAMe is a critical intermediate in numerous reactions in the body. SAMe is a sulfur containing compound that is a critical intermediate in the methylation methionine/folate cycle and also serves as a methyl donor in the body. If this is more methylation than he/she is able to handle, and he/she begins to exhibit mood swings, then you can adjust the balance between the use of methyl and hydroxy B12 to favor more hydroxy B12, and also decrease the dose of SAMe or eliminate it entirely. Conversely, in the future if he/she is tolerating methyl donors well, you can consider the use of other methyl donors. You may want to consider the use of curcumin, melatonin, FgF, theanine, ZEN, and MSM (not for those with CBS C699T + status) in addition to the specific methyl donors already listed (SAMe, methyl B12).

As the level of B12 becomes more in balance following appropriate supplementation to address the methylation cycle mutation it will also help in balancing glutamate and GABA levels. In addition GABA can be added directly. Plain GABA will be tolerated due to the COMT and VDR status. Where he/she is COMT + - he/she should also be able to tolerate, and benefit from low doses of ZEN which contains theanine in addition to GABA, as theanine has methyl groups. There are several other supplements that are very useful for balancing glutamate and GABA; these include taurine, pycnogenol and grape seed extract. These three are included in the general vitamin; however you may want to consider adding in additional amounts of pycnogenol, grape seed extract and taurine (except for no additional taurine for those with a CBS C699T+ mutation) as needed based on behavior especially as there are only very low doses of these in the general vitamin. GABA levels are related to language, as well as to anxiety levels, particularly anxiety in response to low blood sugar.

Lead inhibits a critical enzyme in the pathway for heme synthesis. A block in this pathway creates a build up of an intermediate that competes with GABA. Reduced GABA activity can cause auditory processing issues as well as language problems, and anxiety. In addition, inhibition of this pathway by lead can cause anemia, as well as the inability to make groups that are needed for B12 synthesis. A lack of these groups will exacerbate mutations in methionine synthase and methionine synthase reductase. This again points to the need for added B12 for individuals with mutations in this portion of the methylation cycle as well as the use of supplements to address lead toxicity in the body. The use of weekly baths in Beyond Clean, which contains EDTA should help to address lead toxicity in a very gentle manner that is suitable to most systems. It is also valuable to consider the use of ½ EDTA capsule per day or the use of EDTA chewing gum.

Once the methylation cycle is supplemented properly you may begin to see an increased level of detoxification. Generally there will be a one week "honeymoon" period followed by a regression in behaviors as the creatinine starts to climb. In order to monitor this and to understand changes in behavior that may occur as a result of this detoxification, it is a good idea to take spot urine samples and run urine toxic metal tests. It may seem like a supplement is non ideal for an individual. However, it is difficult to tell the difference between a negative reaction to a supplement and the behavioral impact of detoxification or a mood swing due to dopamine fluxes as the methylation pathway is supplemented properly; that is why use of regular urine toxic metal tests is so critical. The urine samples will help to separate the effects of methylation support on detoxification from supplements that do not agree with an individual.

COMT + + VDR Bsm/Taq - -

- COMT + +   VDR Bsm/Taq - -

    The nutrigenomics report for this individual shows a homozygous mutation in the COMT gene. This means that he/she is COMT + +, and will mean that dopamine levels should be less of an issue for him/her as we look at an overall supplement plan. This will mean that supporting dopamine levels should not play a role in the overall supplement plan. This individual is also VDR Bsm/Taq - - as such he/she will be exquisitely sensitive to methyl donors that are added as part of any supplement plan. While this will mean that dopamine levels may be less of an issue for him/her as you look at an overall supplement plan, it will require caution in the use of methyl donors. On a positive note, he/she will also tend to heal and bounce back much faster than individuals who are COMT - - and should have a lower body burden of toxic metals and chronic viral infections. However, please use caution in the use of methyl donors and pay careful attention to the total amount of methyl donors in the supplement plan as well as to the total amount of dopamine containing foods that are ingested on a given day. Too many methyl donors may cause he/she to have mood swings. Pay careful attention to lithium and iodine levels during any detoxification of heavy metals, as excretion of mercury can affect the levels of lithium and iodine. These essential minerals appear to play an important role in helping to balance mood swings that can occur as a result of dopamine fluxes. These dopamine fluxes are much more of an issue in individuals who are COMT + + regardless of their VDR Bsm and Taq status.

    It is also important to pay attention to foods containing a high level of tyrosine that may increase dopamine levels. Tyrosine and tryptophan will compete with each other for transport into the cell. Tryptophan helps to support serotonin levels and tyrosine helps to support dopamine levels. Therefore it is wise to consider the list of high tryptophan and

high dopamine foods and try to concentrate on more of the high tryptophan foods and to limit the intake of the high tyrosine foods in an effort to support serotonin levels and to prevent mood swings due to dopamine overload.

- COMT + + VDR Bsm/Taq - -
- MTR + or + +

There is also a mutation in the methionine synthase gene (MS or MTR). The methionine synthase mutation is an up regulation mutation that enhances the activity of the enzyme. This should cause the enzyme to use up added B12 at an even faster rate than normal. What this means in practical terms is that he/she may be deficient in methyl B12. The supplementation of B12 is therefore very important for him/her. What will be a bit tricky is to supplement the B12 adequately without causing mood swings due to the COMT + + status. You will want to use hydroxy B12 rather than methyl B12 in an effort to reduce behavioral problems. The balance that has worked well in similar situations in the past is to start with one hydroxy B12 daily. Over the course of a week or two increase the hydroxy B12 first to 2 per day, and then to 3 per day. If you are seeing mood swings, then decrease the hydroxy B12 and move up more slowly in dosage. Literature suggests that oral B12 is as effective as injected B12; however as an alternative you can consider B12 injections. If you decide to use B12 injections it is preferable to use plain hydroxy B12 (no folinic or NAC). If you choose to use B12 injections it may be worth considering the addition of the chewable hydroxy B12 on the injections "off days". If you choose to use injections you can start with injections once a week and gradually increase to injections three times per week. This can be a very gradual process that is dictated by what he/she is able to tolerate; again using chewable B12 on the off days. If you decide to simply use the chewable hydroxy B12 this is an acceptable alternative. You may also want to add sublingual cyano B12 (once a day) to help to support his/her eyes.

As the level of B12 becomes more in balance following appropriate supplementation to address the methionine

synthase mutation it will also help in balancing glutamate and gaba levels. In addition gaba can be added directly. Given the COMT and VDR status the use of plain gaba is suggested rather than ZEN, as the theanine in ZEN contains methyl groups.

There is a second pathway to the formation of methionine through the BHMT enzyme that will bypass this mutation. This pathway uses phosphatidyl serine and /or TMG as donors for the reaction. It is wise to consider adding PS and a small amount of TMG to help to drive this reaction. While DMG works well to support language, it may be best to wait to add any DMG until this pathway is supplemented properly, as the DMG may be inhibiting this BHMT reaction to methionine. Supplementation for this part of the pathway also uses a low dose of TMG, choline and plain methionine. The HHC general vitamin is acceptable as a source for TMG, choline and methionine as well as the other general nutrients contained in it (½-1 in the morning and another ½-1 in the afternoon). In addition, phosphatidyl serine should also be added to help to support the "back door" reaction from homocysteine to methionine via the BHMT enzyme. Phosphatidyl serine is available as plain PS gel caps as well as a chewable form with DMAE (Pedi-Active). DMAE contains methyl groups so the plain PS gel caps are the preferred form of this supplement rather than the chewable form given the COMT and VDR status. If even the use of plain PS seems to be a problem in terms of mood swings or depression then simply use the low doses of the HHC general vitamin. This will help to support the alternative pathway that will bypass the mutations in the MTR gene.

To summarize at this point, due to the COMT and VDR status appropriate methylation supplementation should include ¼ Folapro, ¼ Intrinsic B12, hydroxy B12, ¼ nucleotides, and ¼ dropper Methylation Support RNA, one to two of the HHC general vitamins, and a plain phosphatidyl serine gel cap. If mood swings occur then discontinue the use of phosphatidyl serine, also decrease the dose of hydroxy B12 and decrease the Folapro to 1/8 per day if needed. The biggest issue for him/her will be balancing the need for these methylation supplements, yet at the same time preventing mood swings due to dopamine excess. You will want to avoid the use of additional methyl donors which include curcumin, melatonin, FgF, theanine, ZEN, and MSM, SAMe, and methyl B12.

As the level of B12 becomes more in balance following appropriate methylation cycle supplementation it will also help in balancing glutamate and GABA levels. In addition plain GABA can be added directly. Plain GABA will be tolerated the best due to the COMT and VDR status. Where he/she is COMT + + or COMT + - VDR Bsm/Taq - - he/she will not be able to tolerate ZEN which contains theanine in addition to GABA. There are several other supplements that are very useful for balancing glutamate and GABA; these include taurine, pycnogenol and grape seed extract. These three are included in the general vitamin; however you may want to consider adding in additional amounts of pycnogenol, grape seed extract and taurine (except for no additional taurine for those with a CBS C699T+ mutation) as needed based on behavior especially as there are only very low doses of these in the general vitamin. GABA levels are related to language, as well as to anxiety levels, particularly anxiety in response to low blood sugar.

Lead inhibits a critical enzyme in the pathway for heme synthesis. A block in this pathway creates a build up of an intermediate that competes with GABA. Reduced GABA activity can cause auditory processing issues as well as language problems, and anxiety. In addition, inhibition of this pathway by lead can cause anemia, as well as the inability to make groups that are needed for B12 synthesis. A lack of these groups will exacerbate mutations in methionine synthase and methionine synthase reductase. This again points to the need for added B12 for individuals with mutations in this portion of the methylation cycle as well as the use of supplements to address lead toxicity in the body. The use of weekly baths in Beyond Clean, which contains EDTA should help to address lead toxicity in a very gentle manner that is suitable to most systems. It is also valuable to consider the use of ½ EDTA capsule per day or the use of EDTA chewing gum.

Once the methylation cycle is supplemented properly you may begin to see an increased level of detoxification. Generally there will be a one week "honeymoon" period followed by a regression in behaviors as the creatinine starts to climb. In order to monitor this and to understand changes in behavior that may occur as a result of this detoxification, it is a good idea to take spot urine samples and run urine toxic metal tests. It may seem like a supplement is non ideal for an individual. However, it is difficult to tell the difference between a negative reaction to a supplement and the behavioral impact of detoxification or a mood swing due to dopamine fluxes as the methylation pathway is supplemented properly; that is why use of regular urine toxic metal tests is so critical. The urine samples will help to separate the effects of methylation support on detoxification from supplements that do not agree with an individual.

- COMT + + VDR Bsm/Taq - -
- MTRR + or + +

There is also a mutation in the methionine synthase reductase gene (MS_MTRR or MSR). The function of MSR is to regenerate B12 for the MS to utilize. What this means in practical terms is that he/she may be deficient in methyl B12. The supplementation of B12 is therefore very important for him/her. What will be a bit tricky is to supplement the B12 adequately without causing mood swings due to the COMT + + status. You will want to use hydroxy B12 rather than methyl B12 in an effort to reduce behavioral problems. The balance that has worked well in similar situations in the past is to start with one hydroxy B12 daily. Over the course of a week or two increase the hydroxy B12 first to 2 per day, and then to 3 per day. If you are seeing mood swings, then decrease the hydroxy B12 and move up more slowly in dosage. Literature suggests that oral B12 is as effective as injected B12; however as an alternative you can consider B12 injections. If you decide to use B12 injections it is preferable to use plain hydroxy B12 (no folinic or NAC). If you choose to use B12 injections it may be worth considering the addition of the chewable hydroxy B12 on the injections "off days". If you choose to use injections you can start with injections once a week and gradually increase to injections three times per week. This can be a very gradual process that is dictated by what he/she is able to tolerate; again using chewable B12 on the off days. If you decide to simply use the chewable hydroxy B12 this is an acceptable alternative. You may also want to add sublingual cyano B12 (once a day) to help to support his/her eyes.

As the level of B12 becomes more in balance following appropriate supplementation to address the methionine synthase reductase mutation it will also help in balancing

glutamate and gaba levels. In addition gaba can be added directly. Given the COMT and VDR status the use of plain gaba is suggested rather than ZEN, as the theanine in ZEN contains methyl groups.

There is a second pathway to the formation of methionine through the BHMT enzyme that will bypass this mutation. This pathway uses phosphatidyl serine and /or TMG as donors for the reaction. It is wise to consider adding PS and a small amount of TMG to help to drive this reaction. While DMG works well to support language, it may be best to wait to add any DMG until this pathway is supplemented properly, as the DMG may be inhibiting this BHMT reaction to methionine. Supplementation for this part of the pathway also uses a low dose of TMG, choline and plain methionine. The HHC general vitamin is acceptable as a source for TMG, choline and methionine as well as the other general nutrients contained in it (½-1 in the morning and another ½-1 in the afternoon). In addition, phosphatidyl serine should also be added to help to support the "back door" reaction from homocysteine to methionine via the BHMT enzyme as plain PS gel caps as well as a chewable form with DMAE (Pedi-Active). DMAE contains methyl groups so the plain PS gel caps are the preferred form of this supplement rather than the chewable form given the COMT and VDR status. If even the use of plain PS seems to be a problem in terms of mood swings or depression then simply use the low doses of the HHC general vitamin. This will help to support the alternative pathway that will bypass the mutation in the MS_MTRR gene.

To summarize at this point, due to the COMT and VDR status appropriate methylation supplementation should include ¼ Folapro, ¼ Intrinsic B12, hydroxy B12, ¼ nucleotides, and ¼ dropper Methylation Support RNA, one to two of the HHC general vitamins, and a plain phosphatidyl serine gel cap. If mood swings occur then discontinue the use of phosphatidyl serine, also decrease the dose of hydroxy B12 and decrease the Folapro to 1/8 per day if needed. The biggest issue for him/her will be balancing the need for these methylation supplements, yet at the same time preventing mood swings due to dopamine excess. You will want to avoid the use of additional methyl donors which include curcumin, melatonin, FgF, theanine, ZEN, and MSM, SAMe, and methyl B12.

As the level of B12 becomes more in balance following appropriate methylation cycle supplementation it will also help in balancing glutamate and GABA levels. In addition plain GABA can be added directly. Plain GABA will be tolerated the best due to the COMT and VDR status. Where he/she is COMT + + or COMT + - VDR Bsm/Taq - - he/she will not be able to tolerate ZEN which contains theanine in addition to GABA. There are several other supplements that are very useful for balancing glutamate and GABA; these include taurine, pycnogenol and grape seed extract. These three are included in the general vitamin; however you may want to consider adding in additional amounts of pycnogenol, grape seed extract and taurine (except for no additional taurine for those with a CBS C699T+ mutation) as needed based on behavior especially as there are only very low doses of these in the general vitamin. GABA levels are related to language, as well as to anxiety levels, particularly anxiety in response to low blood sugar.

Lead inhibits a critical enzyme in the pathway for heme synthesis. A block in this pathway creates a build up of an intermediate that competes with GABA. Reduced GABA activity can cause auditory processing issues as well as language problems, and anxiety. In addition, inhibition of this pathway by lead can cause anemia, as well as the inability to make groups that are needed for B12 synthesis. A lack of these groups will exacerbate mutations in methionine synthase and methionine synthase reductase. This again points to the need for added B12 for individuals with mutations in this portion of the methylation cycle as well as the use of supplements to address lead toxicity in the body. The use of weekly baths in Beyond Clean, which contains EDTA should help to address lead toxicity in a very gentle manner that is suitable to most systems. It is also valuable to consider the use of ½ EDTA capsule per day or the use of EDTA chewing gum.

Once the methylation cycle is supplemented properly you may begin to see an increased level of detoxification. Generally there will be a one week "honeymoon" period followed by a regression in behaviors as the creatinine starts to climb. In order to monitor this and to understand changes in behavior that may occur as a result of this detoxification, it is a good idea to take spot urine samples and run urine toxic metal tests. It may seem like a supplement is non ideal for an individual. However, it is difficult to tell the difference between a negative reaction to a supplement and the behavioral impact of detoxification or a mood swing due to dopamine fluxes as the methylation pathway is supplemented properly; that is why use of regular urine toxic metal tests is so critical. The urine samples will help to separate the effects of methylation support on detoxification from supplements that do not agree with an individual.

- COMT + + VDR Bsm/Taq - -
- MTR + or + +
- MTRR + or + +

There is also a mutation in the methionine synthase reductase gene (MS_MTRR or MSR), as well as a mutation in the methionine synthase gene (MS or MTR). The function of MSR is to regenerate B12 for the MS to utilize. The methionine synthase mutation is an up regulation mutation that enhances the activity of the enzyme. This should cause the enzyme to use up added B12 at an even faster rate than normal. What this means in practical terms is that he/she may be severely deficient in methyl B12. The supplementation of B12 is therefore very important for him/her. What will be a bit tricky is to supplement the B12 adequately without causing mood swings due to the COMT + + status. You will want to use hydroxy B12 rather than methyl B12 in an effort to reduce behavioral problems. The balance that has worked well in similar situations in the past is to start with one hydroxy B12 daily. Over the course of a week or two increase the hydroxy B12 first to 2 per day, and then to 3 per day. If you are seeing mood swings, then decrease the hydroxy B12 and move up more slowly in dosage. Literature suggests that oral B12 is as effective as injected B12; however as an alternative you can consider B12 injections. If you decide to use B12 injections it is preferable to use plain hydroxy B12 (no folinic or NAC). If you choose to use B12 injections it may be worth considering the addition of the chewable hydroxy B12 on the injections "off days". If you choose to use injections you can start with injections once a week and gradually increase to injections three times per week. This can be a very gradual process that is dictated by what he/she is able to tolerate; again using chewable B12 on the off days. If you decide to simply use the chewable hydroxy B12 this is an acceptable alternative. You

may also want to add sublingual cyano B12 (once a day) to help to support his/her eyes.

As the level of B12 becomes more in balance following appropriate supplementation to address the methionine synthase reductase mutation and methionine synthase mutations it will also help in balancing glutamate and gaba levels. In addition gaba can be added directly. Given the COMT and VDR status the use of plain gaba is suggested rather than ZEN, as the theanine in ZEN contains methyl groups.

There is a second pathway to the formation of methionine through the BHMT enzyme that will bypass both of these mutations. This pathway uses phosphatidyl serine and /or TMG as donors for the reaction. It is wise to consider adding PS and a small amount of TMG to help to drive this reaction. While DMG works well to support language, it may be best to wait to add any DMG until this pathway is supplemented properly, as the DMG may be inhibiting this BHMT reaction to methionine. Supplementation for this part of the pathway also uses a low dose of TMG, choline and plain methionine. The HHC general vitamin is acceptable as a source for TMG, choline and methionine as well as the other general nutrients contained in it (½-1 in the morning and another ½-1 in the afternoon). In addition, phosphatidyl serine should also be added to help to support the "back door" reaction from homocysteine to methionine via the BHMT enzyme. Phosphatidyl serine is available as plain PS gel caps as well as a chewable form with DMAE (Pedi-Active). DMAE contains methyl groups so the plain PS gel caps are the preferred form of this supplement rather than the chewable form given the COMT and VDR status. If even the use of plain PS seems to be a problem in terms of mood swings or depression then simply use the low doses of the HHC general

vitamin. This will help to support the alternative pathway that will bypass the mutations in the MTR and MS_MTRR genes.

To summarize at this point, due to the COMT and VDR status appropriate methylation supplementation should include ¼ Folapro, ¼ Intrinsic B12, hydroxy B12, ¼ nucleotides, and ¼ dropper Methylation Support RNA, one to two of the HHC general vitamins, and a plain phosphatidyl serine gel cap. If mood swings occur then discontinue the use of phosphatidyl serine, also decrease the dose of hydroxy B12 and decrease the Folapro to 1/8 per day if needed. The biggest issue for him/her will be balancing the need for these methylation supplements, yet at the same time preventing mood swings due to dopamine excess. You will want to avoid the use of additional methyl donors which include curcumin, melatonin, FgF, theanine, ZEN, and MSM, SAMe, and methyl B12.

As the level of B12 becomes more in balance following appropriate methylation cycle supplementation it will also help in balancing glutamate and GABA levels. In addition plain GABA can be added directly. Plain GABA will be tolerated the best due to the COMT and VDR status. Where he/she is COMT + + or COMT + - VDR Bsm/Taq - - he/she will not be able to tolerate ZEN which contains theanine in addition to GABA. There are several other supplements that are very useful for balancing glutamate and GABA; these include taurine, pycnogenol and grape seed extract. These three are included in the general vitamin; however you may want to consider adding in additional amounts of pycnogenol, grape seed extract and taurine (except for no additional taurine for those with a CBS C699T+ mutation) as needed based on behavior especially as there are only very low doses of these in the general vitamin. GABA levels are related to language, as well as to anxiety levels, particularly anxiety in response to low blood sugar.

Lead inhibits a critical enzyme in the pathway for heme synthesis. A block in this pathway creates a build up of an intermediate that competes with GABA. Reduced GABA activity can cause auditory processing issues as well as language problems, and anxiety. In addition, inhibition of this pathway by lead can cause anemia, as well as the inability to make groups that are needed for B12 synthesis. A lack of these groups will exacerbate mutations in methionine synthase and methionine synthase reductase. This again points to the need for added B12 for individuals with mutations in this portion of the methylation cycle as well as the use of supplements to address lead toxicity in the body. The use of weekly baths in Beyond Clean, which contains EDTA should help to address lead toxicity in a very gentle manner that is suitable to most systems. It is also valuable to consider the use of ½ EDTA capsule per day or the use of EDTA chewing gum.

Once the methylation cycle is supplemented properly you may begin to see an increased level of detoxification. Generally there will be a one week "honeymoon" period followed by a regression in behaviors as the creatinine starts to climb. In order to monitor this and to understand changes in behavior that may occur as a result of this detoxification, it is a good idea to take spot urine samples and run urine toxic metal tests. It may seem like a supplement is non ideal for an individual. However, it is difficult to tell the difference between a negative reaction to a supplement and the behavioral impact of detoxification or a mood swing due to dopamine fluxes as the methylation pathway is supplemented properly; that is why use of regular urine toxic metal tests is so critical. The urine samples will help to separate the effects of methylation support on detoxification from supplements that do not agree with an individual.

COMT + + VDR Bsm/Taq + -

- COMT + +   VDR Bsm/Taq + -

The nutrigenomics report for this individual shows a homozygous mutation in the COMT gene. This means that he/she is COMT + +, and will mean that dopamine levels should be less of an issue for him/her as we look at an overall supplement plan. This will mean that supporting dopamine levels should not play a role in the overall supplement plan. This individual is also VDR Bsm/Taq + -; as such he/she will be particularly sensitive to methyl donors that are added as part of any supplement plan. While this will mean that dopamine levels may be less of an issue for him/her as you look at an overall supplement plan, it will require caution in the use of methyl donors. On a positive note, he/she will also tend to heal and bounce back much faster than individuals who are COMT - - and should have a lower body burden of toxic metals and chronic viral infections. However, please use caution in the use of methyl donors and pay careful attention to the total amount of methyl donors in the supplement plan as well as to the total amount of dopamine containing foods that are ingested on a given day. Too many methyl donors may cause he/she to have mood swings. Pay careful attention to lithium and iodine levels during any detoxification of heavy metals, as excretion of mercury can affect the levels of lithium and iodine. These essential minerals appear to play an important role in helping to balance mood swings that can occur as a result of dopamine fluxes. These dopamine fluxes are much more of an issue in individuals who are COMT + + regardless of their VDR Bsm and Taq status.

It is also important to pay attention to foods containing a high level of tyrosine that may increase dopamine levels. Tyrosine and tryptophan will compete with each other for transport into the cell. Tryptophan helps to support serotonin levels and tyrosine helps to support dopamine levels. Therefore it is wise to consider the list of high tryptophan and

high dopamine foods and try to concentrate on more of the high tryptophan foods and to limit the intake of the high tyrosine foods in an effort to support serotonin levels and to prevent mood swings due to dopamine overload.

- COMT + + VDR Bsm/Taq + -
- MTR + or + +

There is also a mutation in the methionine synthase gene (MS or MTR). The methionine synthase mutation is an up regulation mutation that enhances the activity of the enzyme. This should cause the enzyme to use up added B12 at an even faster rate than normal. What this means in practical terms is that he/she may be deficient in methyl B12. The supplementation of B12 is therefore very important for him/her. What will be a bit tricky is to supplement the B12 adequately without causing mood swings due to the COMT + + status. You will want to use hydroxy B12 rather than methyl B12 in an effort to reduce behavioral problems. The balance that has worked well in similar situations in the past is to start with one hydroxy B12 daily. Over the course of a week or two increase the hydroxy B12 first to 2 per day, and then to 3 per day. If you are seeing mood swings, then decrease the hydroxy B12 and move up more slowly in dosage. Literature suggests that oral B12 is as effective as injected B12; however as an alternative you can consider B12 injections. If you decide to use B12 injections it is preferable to use plain hydroxy B12 (no folinic or NAC). If you choose to use B12 injections it may be worth considering the addition of the chewable hydroxy B12 on the injections "off days". If you choose to use injections you can start with injections once a week and gradually increase to injections three times per week. This can be a very gradual process that is dictated by what he/she is able to tolerate; again using chewable B12 on the off days. If you decide to simply use the chewable hydroxy B12 this is an acceptable alternative. You may also want to add sublingual cyano B12 (once a day) to help to support his/her eyes.

As the level of B12 becomes more in balance following appropriate supplementation to address the methionine

synthase mutation it will also help in balancing glutamate and gaba levels. In addition gaba can be added directly. Given the COMT and VDR status the use of plain gaba is suggested rather than ZEN, as the theanine in ZEN contains methyl groups.

There is a second pathway to the formation of methionine through the BHMT enzyme that will bypass this mutation. This pathway uses phosphatidyl serine and /or TMG as donors for the reaction. It is wise to consider adding PS and a small amount of TMG to help to drive this reaction. While DMG works well to support language, it may be best to wait to add any DMG until this pathway is supplemented properly, as the DMG may be inhibiting this BHMT reaction to methionine. Supplementation for this part of the pathway also uses a low dose of TMG, choline and plain methionine. The HHC general vitamin is acceptable as a source for TMG, choline and methionine as well as the other general nutrients contained in it (½-1 in the morning and another ½-1 in the afternoon). In addition, phosphatidyl serine should also be added to help to support the "back door" reaction from homocysteine to methionine via the BHMT enzyme. Phosphatidyl serine is available as plain PS gel caps as well as a chewable form with DMAE (Pedi-Active). DMAE contains methyl groups so the plain PS gel caps are the preferred form of this supplement rather than the chewable form given the COMT and VDR status. If even the use of plain PS seems to be a problem in terms of mood swings or depression then simply use the low doses of the HHC general vitamin. This will help to support the alternative pathway that will bypass the mutations in the MTR gene.

To summarize at this point, due to the COMT and VDR status appropriate methylation supplementation should include ¼ Folapro, ¼ Intrinsic B12, hydroxy B12, ¼ nucleotides, and ¼ dropper Methylation Support RNA, one to two of the HHC general vitamins, and a plain phosphatidyl serine gel cap. If mood swings occur then discontinue the use of phosphatidyl serine, also decrease the dose of hydroxy B12 and decrease the Folapro to 1/8 per day if needed. The biggest issue for him/her will be balancing the need for these methylation supplements, yet at the same time preventing mood swings due to dopamine excess. You will want to avoid the use of additional methyl donors which include curcumin, melatonin, FgF, theanine, ZEN, and MSM, SAMe, and methyl B12.

As the level of B12 becomes more in balance following appropriate methylation cycle supplementation it will also help in balancing glutamate and GABA levels. In addition plain GABA can be added directly. Plain GABA will be tolerated the best due to the COMT and VDR status. Where he/she is COMT + + or COMT + - VDR Bsm/Taq - - he/she will not be able to tolerate ZEN which contains theanine in addition to GABA. There are several other supplements that are very useful for balancing glutamate and GABA; these include taurine, pycnogenol and grape seed extract. These three are included in the general vitamin; however you may want to consider adding in additional amounts of pycnogenol, grape seed extract and taurine (except for no additional taurine for those with a CBS C699T+ mutation) as needed based on behavior especially as there are only very low doses of these in the general vitamin. GABA levels are related to language, as well as to anxiety levels, particularly anxiety in response to low blood sugar.

Lead inhibits a critical enzyme in the pathway for heme synthesis. A block in this pathway creates a build up of an intermediate that competes with GABA. Reduced GABA activity can cause auditory processing issues as well as language problems, and anxiety. In addition, inhibition of this pathway by lead can cause anemia, as well as the inability to make groups that are needed for B12 synthesis. A lack of these groups will exacerbate mutations in methionine synthase and methionine synthase reductase. This again points to the need for added B12 for individuals with mutations in this portion of the methylation cycle as well as the use of supplements to address lead toxicity in the body. The use of weekly baths in Beyond Clean, which contains EDTA should help to address lead toxicity in a very gentle manner that is suitable to most systems. It is also valuable to consider the use of ½ EDTA capsule per day or the use of EDTA chewing gum.

Once the methylation cycle is supplemented properly you may begin to see an increased level of detoxification. Generally there will be a one week "honeymoon" period followed by a regression in behaviors as the creatinine starts to climb. In order to monitor this and to understand changes in behavior that may occur as a result of this detoxification, it is a good idea to take spot urine samples and run urine toxic metal tests. It may seem like a supplement is non ideal for an individual. However, it is difficult to tell the difference between a negative reaction to a supplement and the behavioral impact of detoxification or a mood swing due to dopamine fluxes as the methylation pathway is supplemented properly; that is why use of regular urine toxic metal tests is so critical. The urine samples will help to separate the effects of methylation support on detoxification from supplements that do not agree with an individual.

- COMT + + VDR Bsm/Taq + -
- MTRR + or + +

There is also a mutation in the methionine synthase reductase gene (MS_MTRR or MSR). The function of MSR is to regenerate B12 for the MS to utilize. What this means in practical terms is that he/she may be deficient in methyl B12. The supplementation of B12 is therefore very important for him/her. What will be a bit tricky is to supplement the B12 adequately without causing mood swings due to the COMT + + status. You will want to use hydroxy B12 rather than methyl B12 in an effort to reduce behavioral problems. The balance that has worked well in similar situations in the past is to start with one hydroxy B12 daily. Over the course of a week or two increase the hydroxy B12 first to 2 per day, and then to 3 per day. If you are seeing mood swings, then decrease the hydroxy B12 and move up more slowly in dosage. Literature suggests that oral B12 is as effective as injected B12; however as an alternative you can consider B12 injections. If you decide to use B12 injections it is preferable to use plain hydroxy B12 (no folinic or NAC). If you choose to use B12 injections it may be worth considering the addition of the chewable hydroxy B12 on the injections "off days". If you choose to use injections you can start with injections once a week and gradually increase to injections three times per week. This can be a very gradual process that is dictated by what he/she is able to tolerate; again using chewable B12 on the off days. If you decide to simply use the chewable hydroxy B12 this is an acceptable alternative. You may also want to add sublingual cyano B12 (once a day) to help to support his/her eyes.

As the level of B12 becomes more in balance following appropriate supplementation to address the methionine synthase reductase mutation it will also help in balancing

glutamate and gaba levels. In addition gaba can be added directly. Given the COMT and VDR status the use of plain gaba is suggested rather than ZEN, as the theanine in ZEN contains methyl groups.

There is a second pathway to the formation of methionine through the BHMT enzyme that will bypass this mutation. This pathway uses phosphatidyl serine and /or TMG as donors for the reaction. It is wise to consider adding PS and a small amount of TMG to help to drive this reaction. While DMG works well to support language, it may be best to wait to add any DMG until this pathway is supplemented properly, as the DMG may be inhibiting this BHMT reaction to methionine. Supplementation for this part of the pathway also uses a low dose of TMG, choline and plain methionine. The HHC general vitamin is acceptable as a source for TMG, choline and methionine as well as the other general nutrients contained in it (½-1 in the morning and another ½-1 in the afternoon). In addition, phosphatidyl serine should also be added to help to support the "back door" reaction from homocysteine to methionine via the BHMT enzyme. Phosphatidyl serine is available as plain PS gel caps as well as a chewable form with DMAE (Pedi-Active). DMAE contains methyl groups so the plain PS gel caps are the preferred form of this supplement rather than the chewable form given the COMT and VDR status. If even the use of plain PS seems to be a problem in terms of mood swings or depression then simply use the low doses of the HHC general vitamin. This will help to support the alternative pathway that will bypass the mutation in the MS_MTRR gene.

To summarize at this point, due to the COMT and VDR status appropriate methylation supplementation should include ¼ Folapro, ¼ Intrinsic B12, hydroxy B12, ¼ nucleotides, and ¼ dropper Methylation Support RNA, one to two of the HHC general vitamins, and a plain phosphatidyl

serine gel cap. If mood swings occur then discontinue the use of phosphatidyl serine, also decrease the dose of hydroxy B12 and decrease the Folapro to 1/8 per day if needed. The biggest issue for him/her will be balancing the need for these methylation supplements, yet at the same time preventing mood swings due to dopamine excess. You will want to avoid the use of additional methyl donors which include curcumin, melatonin, FgF, theanine, ZEN, and MSM, SAMe, and methyl B12.

As the level of B12 becomes more in balance following appropriate methylation cycle supplementation it will also help in balancing glutamate and GABA levels. In addition plain GABA can be added directly. Plain GABA will be tolerated the best due to the COMT and VDR status. Where he/she is COMT + + or COMT + - VDR Bsm/Taq - - he/she will not be able to tolerate ZEN which contains theanine in addition to GABA. There are several other supplements that are very useful for balancing glutamate and GABA; these include taurine, pycnogenol and grape seed extract. These three are included in the general vitamin; however you may want to consider adding in additional amounts of pycnogenol, grape seed extract and taurine (except for no additional taurine for those with a CBS C699T+ mutation) as needed based on behavior especially as there are only very low doses of these in the general vitamin. GABA levels are related to language, as well as to anxiety levels, particularly anxiety in response to low blood sugar.

Lead inhibits a critical enzyme in the pathway for heme synthesis. A block in this pathway creates a build up of an intermediate that competes with GABA. Reduced GABA activity can cause auditory processing issues as well as language problems, and anxiety. In addition, inhibition of this pathway by lead can cause anemia, as well as the inability to make groups that are needed for B12 synthesis. A lack of

these groups will exacerbate mutations in methionine synthase and methionine synthase reductase. This again points to the need for added B12 for individuals with mutations in this portion of the methylation cycle as well as the use of supplements to address lead toxicity in the body. The use of weekly baths in Beyond Clean, which contains EDTA should help to address lead toxicity in a very gentle manner that is suitable to most systems. It is also valuable to consider the use of ½ EDTA capsule per day or the use of EDTA chewing gum.

Once the methylation cycle is supplemented properly you may begin to see an increased level of detoxification. Generally there will be a one week "honeymoon" period followed by a regression in behaviors as the creatinine starts to climb. In order to monitor this and to understand changes in behavior that may occur as a result of this detoxification, it is a good idea to take spot urine samples and run urine toxic metal tests. It may seem like a supplement is non ideal for an individual. However, it is difficult to tell the difference between a negative reaction to a supplement and the behavioral impact of detoxification or a mood swing due to dopamine fluxes as the methylation pathway is supplemented properly; that is why use of regular urine toxic metal tests is so critical. The urine samples will help to separate the effects of methylation support on detoxification from supplements that do not agree with an individual.

- COMT + + VDR Bsm/Taq + -
- MTR + or + +
- MTRR + or + +

There is also a mutation in the methionine synthase reductase gene (MS_MTRR or MSR), as well as a mutation in the methionine synthase gene (MS or MTR). The function of MSR is to regenerate B12 for the MS to utilize. The methionine synthase mutation is an up regulation mutation that enhances the activity of the enzyme. This should cause the enzyme to use up added B12 at an even faster rate than normal. What this means in practical terms is that he/she may be severely deficient in methyl B12. The supplementation of B12 is therefore very important for him/her. What will be a bit tricky is to supplement the B12 adequately without causing mood swings due to the COMT + + status. You will want to use hydroxy B12 rather than methyl B12 in an effort to reduce behavioral problems. The balance that has worked well in similar situations in the past is to start with one hydroxy B12 daily. Over the course of a week or two increase the hydroxy B12 first to 2 per day, and then to 3 per day. If you are seeing mood swings, then decrease the hydroxy B12 and move up more slowly in dosage. Literature suggests that oral B12 is as effective as injected B12; however as an alternative you can consider B12 injections. If you decide to use B12 injections it is preferable to use plain hydroxy B12 (no folinic or NAC). If you choose to use B12 injections it may be worth considering the addition of the chewable hydroxy B12 on the injections "off days". If you choose to use injections you can start with injections once a week and gradually increase to injections three times per week. This can be a very gradual process that is dictated by what he/she is able to tolerate; again using chewable B12 on the off days. If you decide to simply use the chewable hydroxy B12 this is an acceptable alternative. You

may also want to add sublingual cyano B12 (once a day) to help to support his/her eyes.

As the level of B12 becomes more in balance following appropriate supplementation to address the methionine synthase reductase mutation and methionine synthase mutations it will also help in balancing glutamate and gaba levels. In addition gaba can be added directly. Given the COMT and VDR status the use of plain gaba is suggested rather than ZEN, as the theanine in ZEN contains methyl groups.

There is a second pathway to the formation of methionine through the BHMT enzyme that will bypass both of these mutations. This pathway uses phosphatidyl serine and /or TMG as donors for the reaction. It is wise to consider adding PS and a small amount of TMG to help to drive this reaction. While DMG works well to support language, it may be best to wait to add any DMG until this pathway is supplemented properly, as the DMG may be inhibiting this BHMT reaction to methionine. Supplementation for this part of the pathway also uses a low dose of TMG, choline and plain methionine. The HHC general vitamin is acceptable as a source for TMG, choline and methionine as well as the other general nutrients contained in it (½-1 in the morning and another ½-1 in the afternoon). In addition, phosphatidyl serine should also be added to help to support the "back door" reaction from homocysteine to methionine via the BHMT enzyme. Phosphatidyl serine is available as plain PS gel caps as well as a chewable form with DMAE (Pedi-Active). DMAE contains methyl groups so the plain PS gel caps are the preferred form of this supplement rather than the chewable form given the COMT and VDR status. If even the use of plain PS seems to be a problem in terms of mood swings or depression then simply use the low doses of the HHC general

vitamin. This will help to support the alternative pathway that will bypass the mutations in the MTR and MS_MTRR genes.

COMT + + VDR Bsm/Taq + +

- COMT + +   VDR Bsm/Taq + +

The nutrigenomics report for this individual shows a homozygous mutation in the COMT gene. This means that he/she is COMT + +, and will mean that dopamine levels should be less of an issue for him/her as we look at an overall supplement plan.. This will mean that supporting dopamine levels should not be an issue as we look at the overall supplement plan. This individual is also homozygous for the VDR Bsm/Taq + +. As such he/she will not be as exquisitely sensitive to methyl donors as individuals who are COMT + + and Bsm/Taq - - and this may allow you a little bit of latitude to use low doses of certain methyl donors as part of a comprehensive supplement plan. What this means in practical terms is that because he/she is COMT + - and VDR Bsm/Taq + - you will be able to use a few more methyl donors in key places in his/her supplement program. However, please use caution in the use of methyl donors and pay careful attention to the total amount of methyl donors in the supplement plan as well as to the total amount of dopamine containing foods that are ingested on a given day. Too many methyl donors may cause he/she to have mood swings. Pay careful attention to lithium and iodine levels during any detoxification of heavy metals, as excretion of mercury can affect the levels of lithium and iodine. These essential minerals appear to play an important role in helping to balance mood swings that can occur as a result of dopamine fluxes. These dopamine fluxes are much more of an issue in individuals who are COMT + + regardless of their VDR Bsm and Taq status.

It is also important to pay attention to foods containing a high level of tyrosine that may increase dopamine levels. Tyrosine and tryptophan will compete with each other for transport into the cell. Tryptophan helps to support serotonin levels and tyrosine helps to support dopamine levels. Therefore it is wise to consider the list of high tryptophan and

high dopamine foods and try to concentrate on more of the high tryptophan foods and to limit the intake of the high tyrosine foods in an effort to support serotonin levels and to prevent mood swings due to dopamine overload.

- COMT + + VDR Bsm/Taq + +
- MTR + or + +

There is also a mutation in the methionine synthase gene (MS or MTR). The methionine synthase mutation is an up regulation mutation that enhances the activity of the enzyme. This should cause the enzyme to use up added B12 at an even faster rate than normal. What this means in practical terms is that he/she may be deficient in methyl B12. The supplementation of B12 is therefore very important for him/her. What will be a bit tricky is to supplement the B12 adequately without causing mood swings due to the COMT + + status. You will want to use hydroxy B12 rather than methyl B12 in an effort to reduce behavioral problems. The balance that has worked well in similar situations in the past is to start with one hydroxy B12 daily. Over the course of a week or two increase the hydroxy B12 first to 2 per day, and then to 3 per day. If you are seeing mood swings, then decrease the hydroxy B12 and move up more slowly in dosage. Literature suggests that oral B12 is as effective as injected B12; however as an alternative you can consider B12 injections. If you decide to use B12 injections it is preferable to use plain hydroxy B12 (no folinic or NAC). If you choose to use B12 injections it may be worth considering the addition of the chewable hydroxy B12 on the injections "off days". If you choose to use injections you can start with injections once a week and gradually increase to injections three times per week. This can be a very gradual process that is dictated by what he/she is able to tolerate; again using chewable B12 on the off days. If you decide to simply use the chewable hydroxy B12 this is an acceptable alternative. You may also want to add sublingual cyano B12 (once a day) to help to support his/her eyes.

As the level of B12 becomes more in balance following appropriate supplementation to address the methionine

synthase mutation it will also help in balancing glutamate and gaba levels. In addition gaba can be added directly. Given the COMT and VDR status the use of plain gaba is suggested rather than ZEN, as the theanine in ZEN contains methyl groups.

There is a second pathway to the formation of methionine through the BHMT enzyme that will bypass this mutation. This pathway uses phosphatidyl serine and /or TMG as donors for the reaction. It is wise to consider adding PS and a small amount of TMG to help to drive this reaction. While DMG works well to support language, it may be best to wait to add any DMG until this pathway is supplemented properly, as the DMG may be inhibiting this BHMT reaction to methionine. Supplementation for this part of the pathway also uses a low dose of TMG, choline and plain methionine. The HHC general vitamin is acceptable as a source for TMG, choline and methionine as well as the other general nutrients contained in it (½-1 in the morning and another ½-1 in the afternoon). In addition, phosphatidyl serine should also be added to help to support the "back door" reaction from homocysteine to methionine via the BHMT enzyme. Phosphatidyl serine is available as plain PS gel caps as well as a chewable form with DMAE (Pedi-Active). DMAE contains methyl groups so the plain PS gel caps are the preferred form of this supplement rather than the chewable form given the COMT and VDR status. If even the use of plain PS seems to be a problem in terms of mood swings or depression then simply use the low doses of the HHC general vitamin. This will help to support the alternative pathway that will bypass the mutations in the MTR gene.

To summarize at this point, due to the COMT and VDR status appropriate methylation supplementation should include ¼ Folapro, ¼ Intrinsic B12, hydroxy B12, ¼ nucleotides, and ¼ dropper Methylation Support RNA, one to two of the HHC general vitamins, and a plain phosphatidyl serine gel cap. If mood swings occur then discontinue the use of phosphatidyl serine, also decrease the dose of hydroxy B12 and decrease the Folapro to 1/8 per day if needed. The biggest issue for him/her will be balancing the need for these methylation supplements, yet at the same time preventing mood swings due to dopamine excess. You will want to avoid the use of additional methyl donors which include curcumin, melatonin, FgF, theanine, ZEN, and MSM, SAMe, and methyl B12.

As the level of B12 becomes more in balance following appropriate methylation cycle supplementation it will also help in balancing glutamate and GABA levels. In addition plain GABA can be added directly. Plain GABA will be tolerated the best due to the COMT and VDR status. Where he/she is COMT + + or COMT + - VDR Bsm/Taq - - he/she will not be able to tolerate ZEN which contains theanine in addition to GABA. There are several other supplements that are very useful for balancing glutamate and GABA; these include taurine, pycnogenol and grape seed extract. These three are included in the general vitamin; however you may want to consider adding in additional amounts of pycnogenol, grape seed extract and taurine (except for no additional taurine for those with a CBS C699T+ mutation) as needed based on behavior especially as there are only very low doses of these in the general vitamin. GABA levels are related to language, as well as to anxiety levels, particularly anxiety in response to low blood sugar.

Lead inhibits a critical enzyme in the pathway for heme synthesis. A block in this pathway creates a build up of an intermediate that competes with GABA. Reduced GABA activity can cause auditory processing issues as well as language problems, and anxiety. In addition, inhibition of this pathway by lead can cause anemia, as well as the inability to make groups that are needed for B12 synthesis. A lack of

these groups will exacerbate mutations in methionine synthase and methionine synthase reductase. This again points to the need for added B12 for individuals with mutations in this portion of the methylation cycle as well as the use of supplements to address lead toxicity in the body. The use of weekly baths in Beyond Clean, which contains EDTA should help to address lead toxicity in a very gentle manner that is suitable to most systems. It is also valuable to consider the use of ½ EDTA capsule per day or the use of EDTA chewing gum.

Once the methylation cycle is supplemented properly you may begin to see an increased level of detoxification. Generally there will be a one week "honeymoon" period followed by a regression in behaviors as the creatinine starts to climb. In order to monitor this and to understand changes in behavior that may occur as a result of this detoxification, it is a good idea to take spot urine samples and run urine toxic metal tests. It may seem like a supplement is non ideal for an individual. However, it is difficult to tell the difference between a negative reaction to a supplement and the behavioral impact of detoxification or a mood swing due to dopamine fluxes as the methylation pathway is supplemented properly; that is why use of regular urine toxic metal tests is so critical. The urine samples will help to separate the effects of methylation support on detoxification from supplements that do not agree with an individual.

- COMT + + VDR Bsm/Taq + +
- MTRR + or + +

    There is also a mutation in the methionine synthase reductase gene (MS_MTRR or MSR). The function of MSR is to regenerate B12 for the MS to utilize. What this means in practical terms is that he/she may be deficient in methyl B12. The supplementation of B12 is therefore very important for him/her. What will be a bit tricky is to supplement the B12 adequately without causing mood swings due to the COMT + + status. You will want to use hydroxy B12 rather than methyl B12 in an effort to reduce behavioral problems. The balance that has worked well in similar situations in the past is to start with one hydroxy B12 daily. Over the course of a week or two increase the hydroxy B12 first to 2 per day, and then to 3 per day. If you are seeing mood swings, then decrease the hydroxy B12 and move up more slowly in dosage. Literature suggests that oral B12 is as effective as injected B12; however as an alternative you can consider B12 injections. If you decide to use B12 injections it is preferable to use plain hydroxy B12 (no folinic or NAC). If you choose to use B12 injections it may be worth considering the addition of the chewable hydroxy B12 on the injections "off days". If you choose to use injections you can start with injections once a week and gradually increase to injections three times per week. This can be a very gradual process that is dictated by what he/she is able to tolerate; again using chewable B12 on the off days. If you decide to simply use the chewable hydroxy B12 this is an acceptable alternative. You may also want to add sublingual cyano B12 (once a day) to help to support his/her eyes.

    As the level of B12 becomes more in balance following appropriate supplementation to address the methionine synthase reductase mutation it will also help in balancing

glutamate and gaba levels. In addition gaba can be added directly. Given the COMT and VDR status the use of plain gaba is suggested rather than ZEN, as the theanine in ZEN contains methyl groups.

There is a second pathway to the formation of methionine through the BHMT enzyme that will bypass this mutation. This pathway uses phosphatidyl serine and /or TMG as donors for the reaction. It is wise to consider adding PS and a small amount of TMG to help to drive this reaction. While DMG works well to support language, it may be best to wait to add any DMG until this pathway is supplemented properly, as the DMG may be inhibiting this BHMT reaction to methionine. Supplementation for this part of the pathway also uses a low dose of TMG, choline and plain methionine. The HHC general vitamin is acceptable as a source for TMG, choline and methionine as well as the other general nutrients contained in it (½-1 in the morning and another ½-1 in the afternoon). In addition, phosphatidyl serine should also be added to help to support the "back door" reaction from homocysteine to methionine via the BHMT enzyme. Phosphatidyl serine is available as plain PS gel caps as well as a chewable form with DMAE (Pedi-Active). DMAE contains methyl groups so the plain PS gel caps are the preferred form of this supplement rather than the chewable form given the COMT and VDR status. If even the use of plain PS seems to be a problem in terms of mood swings or depression then simply use the low doses of the HHC general vitamin. This will help to support the alternative pathway that will bypass the mutation in the MS_MTRR gene.

To summarize at this point, due to the COMT and VDR status appropriate methylation supplementation should include ¼ Folapro, ¼ Intrinsic B12, hydroxy B12, ¼ nucleotides, and ¼ dropper Methylation Support RNA, one to two of the HHC general vitamins, and a plain phosphatidyl

serine gel cap. If mood swings occur then discontinue the use of phosphatidyl serine, also decrease the dose of hydroxy B12 and decrease the Folapro to 1/8 per day if needed. The biggest issue for him/her will be balancing the need for these methylation supplements, yet at the same time preventing mood swings due to dopamine excess. You will want to avoid the use of additional methyl donors which include curcumin, melatonin, FgF, theanine, ZEN, and MSM, SAMe, and methyl B12.

As the level of B12 becomes more in balance following appropriate methylation cycle supplementation it will also help in balancing glutamate and GABA levels. In addition plain GABA can be added directly. Plain GABA will be tolerated the best due to the COMT and VDR status. Where he/she is COMT + + or COMT + - VDR Bsm/Taq - - he/she will not be able to tolerate ZEN which contains theanine in addition to GABA. There are several other supplements that are very useful for balancing glutamate and GABA; these include taurine, pycnogenol and grape seed extract. These three are included in the general vitamin; however you may want to consider adding in additional amounts of pycnogenol, grape seed extract and taurine (except for no additional taurine for those with a CBS C699T+ mutation) as needed based on behavior especially as there are only very low doses of these in the general vitamin. GABA levels are related to language, as well as to anxiety levels, particularly anxiety in response to low blood sugar.

Lead inhibits a critical enzyme in the pathway for heme synthesis. A block in this pathway creates a build up of an intermediate that competes with GABA. Reduced GABA activity can cause auditory processing issues as well as language problems, and anxiety. In addition, inhibition of this pathway by lead can cause anemia, as well as the inability to make groups that are needed for B12 synthesis. A lack of

these groups will exacerbate mutations in methionine synthase and methionine synthase reductase. This again points to the need for added B12 for individuals with mutations in this portion of the methylation cycle as well as the use of supplements to address lead toxicity in the body. The use of weekly baths in Beyond Clean, which contains EDTA should help to address lead toxicity in a very gentle manner that is suitable to most systems. It is also valuable to consider the use of ½ EDTA capsule per day or the use of EDTA chewing gum.

Once the methylation cycle is supplemented properly you may begin to see an increased level of detoxification. Generally there will be a one week "honeymoon" period followed by a regression in behaviors as the creatinine starts to climb. In order to monitor this and to understand changes in behavior that may occur as a result of this detoxification, it is a good idea to take spot urine samples and run urine toxic metal tests. It may seem like a supplement is non ideal for an individual. However, it is difficult to tell the difference between a negative reaction to a supplement and the behavioral impact of detoxification or a mood swing due to dopamine fluxes as the methylation pathway is supplemented properly; that is why use of regular urine toxic metal tests is so critical. The urine samples will help to separate the effects of methylation support on detoxification from supplements that do not agree with an individual.

- COMT + + VDR Bsm/Taq + +
- MTR + or + +
- MTRR + or + +

There is also a mutation in the methionine synthase reductase gene (MS_MTRR or MSR), as well as a mutation in the methionine synthase gene (MS or MTR). The function of MSR is to regenerate B12 for the MS to utilize. The methionine synthase mutation is an up regulation mutation that enhances the activity of the enzyme. This should cause the enzyme to use up added B12 at an even faster rate than normal. What this means in practical terms is that he/she may be severely deficient in methyl B12. The supplementation of B12 is therefore very important for him/her. What will be a bit tricky is to supplement the B12 adequately without causing mood swings due to the COMT + + status. You will want to use hydroxy B12 rather than methyl B12 in an effort to reduce behavioral problems. The balance that has worked well in similar situations in the past is to start with one hydroxy B12 daily. Over the course of a week or two increase the hydroxy B12 first to 2 per day, and then to 3 per day. If you are seeing mood swings, then decrease the hydroxy B12 and move up more slowly in dosage. Literature suggests that oral B12 is as effective as injected B12; however as an alternative you can consider B12 injections. If you decide to use B12 injections it is preferable to use plain hydroxy B12 (no folinic or NAC). If you choose to use B12 injections it may be worth considering the addition of the chewable hydroxy B12 on the injections "off days". If you choose to use injections you can start with injections once a week and gradually increase to injections three times per week. This can be a very gradual process that is dictated by what he/she is able to tolerate; again using chewable B12 on the off days. If you decide to simply use the chewable hydroxy B12 this is an acceptable alternative. You

may also want to add sublingual cyano B12 (once a day) to help to support his/her eyes.

As the level of B12 becomes more in balance following appropriate supplementation to address the methionine synthase reductase mutation and methionine synthase mutations it will also help in balancing glutamate and gaba levels. In addition gaba can be added directly. Given the COMT and VDR status the use of plain gaba is suggested rather than ZEN, as the theanine in ZEN contains methyl groups.

There is a second pathway to the formation of methionine through the BHMT enzyme that will bypass both of these mutations. This pathway uses phosphatidyl serine and /or TMG as donors for the reaction. It is wise to consider adding PS and a small amount of TMG to help to drive this reaction. While DMG works well to support language, it may be best to wait to add any DMG until this pathway is supplemented properly, as the DMG may be inhibiting this BHMT reaction to methionine. Supplementation for this part of the pathway also uses a low dose of TMG, choline and plain methionine. The HHC general vitamin is acceptable as a source for TMG, choline and methionine as well as the other general nutrients contained in it (½-1 in the morning and another ½-1 in the afternoon). In addition, phosphatidyl serine should also be added to help to support the "back door" reaction from homocysteine to methionine via the BHMT enzyme. Phosphatidyl serine is available as plain PS gel caps as well as a chewable form with DMAE (Pedi-Active). DMAE contains methyl groups so the plain PS gel caps are the preferred form of this supplement rather than the chewable form given the COMT and VDR status. If even the use of plain PS seems to be a problem in terms of mood swings or depression then simply use the low doses of the HHC general

vitamin. This will help to support the alternative pathway that will bypass the mutations in the MTR and MS_MTRR genes.

To summarize at this point, due to the COMT and VDR status appropriate methylation supplementation should include ¼ Folapro, ¼ Intrinsic B12, hydroxy B12, ¼ nucleotides, and ¼ dropper Methylation Support RNA, one to two of the HHC general vitamins, and a plain phosphatidyl serine gel cap. If mood swings occur then discontinue the use of phosphatidyl serine, also decrease the dose of hydroxy B12 and decrease the Folapro to 1/8 per day if needed. The biggest issue for him/her will be balancing the need for these methylation supplements, yet at the same time preventing mood swings due to dopamine excess. You will want to avoid the use of additional methyl donors which include curcumin, melatonin, FgF, theanine, ZEN, and MSM, SAMe, and methyl B12.

As the level of B12 becomes more in balance following appropriate methylation cycle supplementation it will also help in balancing glutamate and GABA levels. In addition plain GABA can be added directly. Plain GABA will be tolerated the best due to the COMT and VDR status. Where he/she is COMT + + or COMT + - VDR Bsm/Taq - - he/she will not be able to tolerate ZEN which contains theanine in addition to GABA. There are several other supplements that are very useful for balancing glutamate and GABA; these include taurine, pycnogenol and grape seed extract. These three are included in the general vitamin; however you may want to consider adding in additional amounts of pycnogenol, grape seed extract and taurine (except for no additional taurine for those with a CBS C699T+ mutation) as needed based on behavior especially as there are only very low doses of these in the general vitamin. GABA levels are related to language, as well as to anxiety levels, particularly anxiety in response to low blood sugar.

Lead inhibits a critical enzyme in the pathway for heme synthesis. A block in this pathway creates a build up of an intermediate that competes with GABA. Reduced GABA activity can cause auditory processing issues as well as language problems, and anxiety. In addition, inhibition of this pathway by lead can cause anemia, as well as the inability to make groups that are needed for B12 synthesis. A lack of these groups will exacerbate mutations in methionine synthase and methionine synthase reductase. This again points to the need for added B12 for individuals with mutations in this portion of the methylation cycle as well as the use of supplements to address lead toxicity in the body. The use of weekly baths in Beyond Clean, which contains EDTA should help to address lead toxicity in a very gentle manner that is suitable to most systems. It is also valuable to consider the use of ½ EDTA capsule per day or the use of EDTA chewing gum.

Once the methylation cycle is supplemented properly you may begin to see an increased level of detoxification. Generally there will be a one week "honeymoon" period followed by a regression in behaviors as the creatinine starts to climb. In order to monitor this and to understand changes in behavior that may occur as a result of this detoxification, it is a good idea to take spot urine samples and run urine toxic metal tests. It may seem like a supplement is non ideal for an individual. However, it is difficult to tell the difference between a negative reaction to a supplement and the behavioral impact of detoxification or a mood swing due to dopamine fluxes as the methylation pathway is supplemented properly; that is why use of regular urine toxic metal tests is so critical. The urine samples will help to separate the effects of methylation support on detoxification from supplements that do not agree with an individual.

MTHFR A1298C

- MTHFR A1298C + or + +

The nutrigenomics test also shows a single A1298C mutation in the MTHFR gene for this individual. This mutation in the MTHFR gene can impact the levels of BH4. The A1298C mutation has been mapped to the SAMe regulatory region of the gene. Mutations in the A1298C do <u>not</u> lead to increased levels of homocysteine; until now it has been felt that this mutation may not be of serious consequence. Literature suggests that the MTHFR enzyme can drive the reverse reaction leading to formation of BH4. I believe that the A1289C mutation is associated with a defect in this reverse reaction leading to the formation of BH4. The A1298C mutation would then be associated with an inability to convert BH2 to BH4 and may cause exceedingly low BH4 levels. This in turn will affect dopamine levels as well as the levels of serotonin and urea cycle function. The COMT and VDR Bsm/Taq status will play a role in affecting overall BH4 levels as any needed synthesis of dopamine to replenish dopamine stores will require BH4. Individuals who are COMT + + or VDR Bsm/Taq - - have an advantage in this area and the COMT + + and VDR Bsm/Taq status will help to compensate to a certain extent for the effect of the MTHFR A1298C mutation. MTHFR A1298C mutations limit the supply of BH4. Low levels of BH4 are also associated with more severe parasitic infections, diabetes as well as hypertension and arteriosclerosis. Serotonin synthesis as well as ammonia detoxification also require BH4. Factors that lead to more ammonia, such as high protein diets, generate more ammonia that needs to be detoxified. Elevated levels of ammonia are sufficient to cause flapping and other over stimulatory behaviors. Excess ammonia in the gut may alter the local pH and aggravate imbalances in microbial flora. Each molecule of ammonia requires two molecules of BH4 for ideal detoxification. It is clear to see how several of these factors may act together to impact ammonia detoxification as well as optimal BH4 levels for neurotransmitter synthesis. Keeping the ammonia levels under control is of paramount importance for overall health and wellness, especially for an individual with an MTHFR A1298C mutation as any excess ammonia generated can drain stores of BH4. This will impact upon serotonin levels and to a certain extent cause fluxes in dopamine (which translates into mood swings). Also helping to restore adequate levels of BH4 should aid in serotonin synthesis, maintaining dopamine levels in a more stable manner as well as ammonia detoxification.

- MTHFR A1298C + or + +
- MTR - -
- MTRR - -

We are fortunate in that he/she does not have mutations in the methionine synthase or the methionine synthase reductase genes. This would suggest that that he/she should not be severely depleted in methyl B12 once the MTHFR A1298C mutation is adequately addressed. As part of a comprehensive program it would still be wise to supplement with some B12; however, high levels of supplementation should not be necessary as he/she does not have mutations in this specific aspect of the pathway. Individuals who are COMT + + should use hydroxy B12 for supplementation, where as those who are more limited in methyl groups due to their COMT VDR status should use methyl B12.

There is a second pathway to the formation of methionine through the BHMT enzyme that will bypass mutations in the methionine synthase and methionine synthase reductase genes. Again, as with the supplementation with B12, it is advisable to support these pathways, however high level supplementation should not be necessary as there are no mutations that have been noted on the nutrigenomic test in the ability to utilize and regenerate methyl B12. This pathway uses phosphatidyl serine and /or TMG as donors for the reaction. It is wise to consider adding PS and a small amount of TMG to help to drive this reaction. While DMG works well to support language, it may be best to wait to add any DMG until this pathway is supplemented properly as the DMG may be inhibiting this BHMT reaction to methionine. Supplementation for this part of the pathway also uses a low dose of TMG, choline and plain methionine. The HHC general vitamin is acceptable as a source for TMG, choline and methionine as well as the other general nutrients contained in it (½-1 in the morning and another ½-1 in the afternoon). In addition, phosphatidyl serine should also be added to help to support the "back door" reaction from homocysteine to methionine via the BHMT enzyme. Phosphatidyl serine is available as plain PS gel caps as well as a chewable form with DMAE (Pedi-Active). DMAE contains methyl groups so this is an ideal form for individuals who need extra methyl groups based on their COMT and VDR test results. Plain phosphatidyl serine is often available as a gelcap and this is a preferred form. Individuals who are COMT ++ should use only the plain phosphatidyl serine gelcaps. Those in need of additional methyl groups due to their COMT and VDR status should consider using one phosphatidyl serine gelcap as well as one of the chewable Pedi-Active PS with DMAE daily.

Individuals should also be supporting the rest of the methylation pathway with ¼ Folapro, ¼ Intrinsic B12, ¼ nucleotides, ¼ dropper methylation support RNA, as well as appropriate support for the CBS up regulation and for the BHMT reaction described above.

MTHFR C677T

- MTHFR C677T + or + +

The nutrigenomics test also shows a single C677T mutation in the MTHFR gene for this individual. While I find this to be the less severe mutation from the standpoint of autism, it does impact the ability of the body to convert homocysteine to methionine. C677T mutations in the MTHFR gene will therefore lead to increased levels of homocysteine if the body is not supplemented properly to address this mutation. High levels of homocysteine have been mentioned in association with heart disease, Alzheimer's disease as well as a range of inflammatory conditions. Homocysteine also serves a regulatory function in the body.

Conditions of high homocysteine favor the accumulation of S adenosyl homocysteine (SAH) in the body. SAH inhibits the activity of several enzymes in the methylation pathway including the inhibition of COMT. While this may offer certain advantages in terms of increasing dopamine levels for individuals who are COMT - -, this inhibition of COMT may create mood swings for COMT + + individuals.

SAH also inhibits enzymes that transfer methyl groups to DNA, RNA and proteins. High levels of homocysteine due to primary mutations in the methylation pathway (i.e. MTHFR C677T) may create secondary problems in this pathway due to inhibition of DNA methylation. Support with appropriate supplementation to address all aspects of the methylation pathway should help to alleviate these effects. Because the C677T mutation in the MTHFR is a mutation in the forward reaction of this enzyme it means that the body is less able to make 5 methyl folate and requires supplementation with this form of folate.

Following appropriate supplementation to address the MTHFR C677T mutation as well as any other mutations in the methylation cycle there will generally be a one week "honeymoon" period followed by a regression in behaviors as the creatinine starts to climb. However, this honeymoon period may be as short as a day for individuals with a C677T mutation, combined with methionine synthase and methionine synthase reductase mutations. This combination of mutations are in such a pivotal location in the methylation cycle, that as soon as you begin to supplement properly, you may see an almost immediate effect on detoxification as this pathway is rapidly unblocked. It may be visualized as if you are suddenly opening the dike on a dam. In order to monitor this and to understand changes in behavior that may occur as a result of this detoxification, you should run spot urine toxic metal tests. It may seem like a supplement is non ideal for an individual. However, it is difficult to tell the difference between a negative reaction to a supplement and the behavioral impact of detoxification or a mood swing due to dopamine fluxes as the methylation pathway is supplemented properly. That is why the regular urine samples are so critical.

- MTHFR C677T + or + +
- MTR - -
- MTRR - -

We are fortunate in that he/she does not have mutations in the methionine synthase or the methionine synthase reductase genes. This would suggest that that he/she should not be severely depleted in methyl B12 once the MTHFR C677T mutation is adequately addressed. As part of a comprehensive program it would still be wise to supplement with some B12; however, high levels of supplementation should not be necessary as he/she does not have mutations in this specific aspect of the pathway. Individuals who are COMT + + should use hydroxy B12 for supplementation where as those who are more limited in methyl groups due to their COMT VDR status should use methyl B12.

There is a second pathway to the formation of methionine through the BHMT enzyme that will bypass mutations in the methionine synthase and methionine synthase reductase genes. Again, as with the supplementation with B12, it is advisable to support these pathways. However, high level supplementation should not be necessary as there are no mutations that have been noted on the nutrigenomic test in the ability to utilize and regenerate methyl B12. This pathway uses phosphatidyl serine and /or TMG as donors for the reaction. It is wise to consider adding PS and a small amount of TMG to help to drive this reaction. While DMG works well to support language, it may be best to wait to add any DMG until this pathway is supplemented properly, as the DMG may be inhibiting this BHMT reaction to methionine.
Supplementation for this part of the pathway also uses a low dose of TMG, choline and plain methionine. The HHC general vitamin is acceptable as a source for TMG, choline and methionine as well as the other general nutrients contained in

it (½-1 in the morning and another ½-1 in the afternoon). In addition, phosphatidyl serine should also be added to help to support the "back door" reaction from homocysteine to methionine via the BHMT enzyme. Phosphatidyl serine is available as plain PS gel caps as well as a chewable form with DMAE (Pedi-Active). DMAE contains methyl groups so this is an ideal form for individuals who need extra methyl groups based on their COMT and VDR test results. Plain phosphatidyl serine is often available as a gelcap and this is a preferred form. Individuals who are COMT ++ should use only the plain phosphatidyl serine gelcaps. Those in need of additional methyl groups due to their COMT and VDR status should consider using one phosphatidyl serine gelcap as well as one of the chewable Pedi-Active PS with DMAE daily.

Individuals should also be supporting the rest of the methylation pathway with ¼ Folapro, ¼ Intrinsic B12, ¼ nucleotides, ¼ dropper methylation support RNA, as well as appropriate support for the CBS up regulation and for the BHMT reaction described above.

CBS C699T

- CBS C699T + or + +

One of the biggest issues for this individual in the methylation cycle is the heterozygous CBS C699T mutation. This mutation will allow for any added methylation cycle supplements to be depleted through the transulfuration pathway to generate additional ammonia and excess sulfur compounds. This creates a "catch 22". It is important to supplement the methylation cycle in order to address viral infection in the body, toxic metal burdens as well as to support neurotransmitters and immune function and myelination of nerves. On the other hand, until the CBS up regulation is under control, there is a risk of any added methylation cycle support creating additional problems in the body. The added ammonia that is generated due to enhanced breakdown of methylation cycle intermediates will put a burden on the urea cycle and will deplete BH4 that is needed for serotonin, dopamine, conversion of phenylalanine to tyrosine and language related function. The excess sulfur can trigger the stress/cortisol response in the body as well as potentially causing a decrease in the enzyme glucose 6 phosphate dehydrogenase (G6PDH).

Fortunately this individual does not have a A1298C mutation in the MTHFR gene which can further impact the levels of BH4. The A1298C mutation has been mapped to the SAMe regulatory region of the gene. Mutations in the A1298C do not lead to increased levels of homocysteine. Until now it has been felt that this mutation may not be of serious consequence. Literature suggests that the MTHFR enzyme can drive the reverse reaction leading to formation of BH4. I believe that the A1289C mutation is associated with a defect in this reverse reaction leading to the formation of BH4. The A1298C mutation would then be associated with an inability to convert BH2 to BH4. Between these two mutations (CBS

C699T and MTHFR A1298C) it may cause exceedingly low BH4 levels. This in turn will affect dopamine levels as well as the levels of serotonin and urea cycle function. The COMT and VDR Bsm/Taq status will play a role in affecting overall BH4 levels as any needed synthesis of dopamine to replenish dopamine stores will require BH4. Individuals who are COMT + + or VDR Bsm/Taq - - have an advantage in this area; the COMT + + and VDR Bsm/Taq status will help to compensate to a certain extent for the effect of the MTHFR A1298C mutation. MTHFR A1298C mutations limit the supply of BH4. Low levels of BH4 are also associated with more severe parasitic infections, diabetes as well as hypertension and arteriosclerosis. Serotonin synthesis as well as ammonia detoxification also require BH4. The CBS C699T leads to more ammonia that needs to be detoxified. Elevated levels of ammonia are sufficient to cause flapping and other over stimulatory behaviors. Excess ammonia in the gut may alter the local pH and aggravate imbalances in microbial flora. Each molecule of ammonia requires two molecules of BH4 for ideal detoxification. It is clear to see how several of these mutations may act together to impact ammonia detoxification as well as optimal BH4 levels for neurotransmitter synthesis. Keeping the CBS C699T+ mutation under control is of paramount importance for overall health and wellness. Any excess ammonia generated by the CBS C699T+ mutation can drain stores of BH4. This will impact upon serotonin levels and to a certain extent cause fluxes in dopamine (which translates into mood swings). Therefore keeping the CBS C699T+ mutation under control is of paramount importance to getting the body back in balance. Also helping to restore adequate levels of BH4 should aid in serotonin synthesis, maintaining dopamine levels in a more stable manner, as well as ammonia detoxification.

In order to address the CBS C699T, it has been found that the use of a low protein diet, in conjunction with ammonia support RNA (1/2 dropper given with methylation cycle supplements and with every meal) will help to balance the system. It will make a big difference if protein in the diet is limited to those foods that will help to support healthy neurotransmitter levels. As discussed above, the balance of high tyrosine and high tryptophan foods should be decided based upon the COMT and VDR Bsm/Taq status. In addition the nightly use of charcoal as a supplement just before bed has proven to aid in controlling excess ammonia levels. The best time for the use of charcoal is just prior to bed to separate the time frame of the addition of the charcoal from other supporting supplements. This should limit the ability to of the charcoal to deplete the body of needed nutrients. It is important to be sure that the bowels are moving well with the addition of charcoal. The use of a magnesium citrate flush (high doses of magnesium citrate) following the addition of 1 to 2 charcoal capsules helps to ensure a bowel movement after this addition of charcoal to soak up excess ammonia. In addition the herb Yucca is reported to aid in ammonia support. The suggested starting dosage is ½ Yucca capsule per day.

A source of low dose P5P rather than a high dose B6 supplement is useful to support the body's B6 requiring reactions and at the same time, not acting to push the CBS reaction. The HHC Neurological Health general vitamin is a very good source of P5P and the other Bs for individuals with CBS C699T mutations in spite of the fact that it does have low concentrations of sulfur containing compounds. It is a bit of a "catch 22"; the body does need the sulfur compounds such as glutathione, but it creates more difficulties when they are added until the CBS mutation has been addressed from a nutritional standpoint. These supplements should help to deal with both aspects of this issue.

The CBS C699T mutation will not only deplete the intermediates in the methylation cycle, it will also lead to elevated levels of taurine and excess sulfur groups. It is recommend that individuals with a CBS C699T+ mutation do not use high levels of taurine or additional sulfur donors (broccoli, etc) as it may create problems with excess sulfur groups (a small amount in a general vitamin is okay but using 500mg taurine capsules is not recommended).

    The CBS C699T mutation will also cause a depletion of molybdenum levels as molybdenum is involved in making sulfur groups less toxic in the body as it is a cofactor for the enzyme sulfite oxidase. Increased amounts of molybdenum may be utilized in individuals with a CBS C699T up regulation in response to the increased generation of sulfur groups via the transulfuration reaction. It may be hard to keep molybdenum in the normal range; this may account in part for copper/ zinc imbalances that are observed as the molybdenum cannot keep up. It is worth running an essential mineral urine test to be certain that molybdenum levels are in the normal range. If not, it would make sense to consider using molybdenum supplementation. The E lyte molybdenum is an easily absorbed source of this mineral. On a related note, xanthine oxidase is another molybdenum requiring enzyme in the body. When milk and other dairy products are not homogenized, components of the milk are digested in the stomach and the small intestine, including the enzyme xanthine oxidase. However, when milk is homogenized, its xanthine oxidase is not broken down, but instead passes into the circulation. The elevated presence of xanthine oxidase may exacerbate limited molybdenum levels and add to further imbalances in the copper levels. This would also suggest that it is wise to continue with a casein free diet and that if you are going to use any dairy products that it may be beneficial to use whole dairy products that are not homogenized particularly for individuals with CBS C699T mutations. Molybdenum, EDTA, carnosine and zinc will help to keep copper/zinc ratios more balanced. Chewable zinc tablets with slippery elm will benefit the gut as well as providing a well controlled dose of zinc. Dosing can start with ¼ tablet and increase to 1 whole tablet per day. The E lyte zinc is an acceptable alternative. BioNativius trace minerals are useful for providing general mineral support along with additional support as needed from the E lyte zinc, molybdenum and magnesium. Essential mineral tests can be run from urine samples to verify that minerals are within range. Pay careful attention to lithium and iodine levels during any detoxification of heavy metals as excretion of mercury can affect the levels of lithium and iodine. These essential minerals appear to play an important role in helping to balance mood swings that can occur as a result of dopamine fluxes. These dopamine fluxes are much more of an issue in individuals who are COMT + + regardless of their VDR Bsm and Taq status. If lithium of lithium or iodine levels are low, useful supplements to support healthy levels include lithium oratate and iodoral. A suggested starting dose is ¼ of capsule/tablet each daily.

A further result of the CBS C699T+ mutation there may be high taurine and very low levels of homocysteine on a urine amino acid test. Individuals with this mutation also tend to have more difficulties with sulfur containing compounds. This would include garlic, broccoli, taurine, glutathione, and even DMPS and DMSA. Once the body is supported nutritionally to address the CBS mutation these individuals are in a better position to be able to use sulfur containing compounds including glutathione.

The CBS C699T will also put some strain on the urea cycle. The availability of BH4 helps to determine whether nitric oxide, peroxy nitrite or super oxide are formed as a function of the urea cycle. Two molecules of BH4 are required for formation of nitric oxide; one molecule of BH4 leads to the formation of peroxy nitrite and the absence of BH4 leads to super oxide formation. The BH4 acts in concert with the NOS enzyme in the urea cycle to produce these end products. There is some literature to suggest that omega 3 EFAs may limit the activity of NOS. As with most other supplements this suggests that moderation is the best approach. The use of an EFA mixture that has omega 3:6:9 every other day, alternating it with a source of omega 3 fatty acids such as DHA should help to strike a reasonable balance in individuals with NOS mutations. For those individuals who do not have NOS mutations, the daily use of an omega 3 mixture in addition to the daily use of a separate source of omega 3s should be fine. In this way the body is supported for optimal membrane fluidity yet at the same time is limiting any negative effects of too much omega 3 on the NOS enzyme. A lower protein diet and the use of Stress RNA once or twice daily will also help to take some of the strain off of the urea cycle. A strain on the urea cycle due to inefficient NOS activity can lead to elevated levels of ammonia that can exacerbate the ammonia problem as a result of the CBS C699T+ mutations and lead to further drains on the already limited stores of BH4.

Preliminary collaborative research is ongoing between myself and a group of doctors in Japan, looking at the use of prescription BH4 to help to compensate for MTHFR A1298C and CBS C699T+ mutations. The initial results in this area are encouraging. Low daily doses of BH4 initially appear to stimulate detoxification over the first several weeks of use. After this initial detoxification effect the BH4 appears to have a very positive impact on language for individuals with CBS C699T+ mutations.

In addition to addressing the CBS C699T mutation, it is important to supplement the methylation pathway to ensure that there are adequate methyl and sulfur donors for the body. Once the CBS up regulation has been addressed, individuals are in a better position to maintain appropriate levels of intermediates in the pathway once they have been added to his/her system rather than having them drain through the CBS C699T which is currently acting like a "hole in the bucket".

- CBS C699T+ or + +
- MTHFR A1298C + or + +

One of the biggest issues in the methylation cycle is the heterozygous CBS C699T mutation. This mutation will allow for any added methylation cycle supplements to be depleted through the transulfuration pathway to generate additional ammonia and excess sulfur compounds. This creates a "catch 22". It is important to supplement the methylation cycle in order to address viral infection in the body, toxic metal burdens, as well as to support neurotransmitters and immune function and myelination of nerves. On the other hand, until the CBS up regulation is under control there is a risk of any added methylation cycle support creating additional problems in the body. The added ammonia that is generated due to enhanced breakdown of methylation cycle intermediates will put a burden on the urea cycle and will deplete BH4 that is needed for serotonin, dopamine, conversion of phenylalanine to tyrosine and language related function. The excess sulfur can trigger the stress/cortisol response in the body as well as potentially causing a decrease in the enzyme glucose 6 phosphate dehydrogenase (G6PDH).

This individual also has a A1298C mutation in the MTHFR gene which may further impact the levels of BH4. The A1298C mutation has been mapped to the SAMe regulatory region of the gene. Mutations in the A1298C do not lead to increased levels of homocysteine. Until now it has been felt that this mutation may not be of serious consequence. Literature suggests that the MTHFR enzyme can drive the reverse reaction leading to formation of BH4. I believe that the A1289C mutation is associated with a defect in this reverse reaction leading to the formation of BH4. The A1298C mutation would then be associated with an inability to convert BH2 to BH4. Between these two mutations (CBS C699T and

MTHFR A1298C) it may cause exceedingly low BH4 levels. This in turn will affect dopamine levels as well as the levels of serotonin and urea cycle function. The COMT and VDR Bsm/Taq status will play a role in affecting overall BH4 levels as any needed synthesis of dopamine to replenish dopamine stores will require BH4. Individuals who are COMT + + or VDR Bsm/Taq - - have an advantage in this area, and the COMT + + and VDR Bsm/Taq status will help to compensate to a certain extent for the effect of the MTHFR A1298C mutation. MTHFR A1298C mutations limit the supply of BH4. Low levels of BH4 are also associated with more severe parasitic infections, diabetes as well as hypertension and arteriosclerosis. Serotonin synthesis as well as ammonia detoxification also require BH4. The CBS C699T leads to more ammonia that needs to be detoxified. Elevated levels of ammonia are sufficient to cause flapping and other over stimulatory behaviors. Excess ammonia in the gut may alter the local pH and aggravate imbalances in microbial flora. Each molecule of ammonia requires two molecules of BH4 for ideal detoxification. It is clear to see how several of these mutations may act together to impact ammonia detoxification as well as optimal BH4 levels for neurotransmitter synthesis. Keeping the CBS C699T+ mutation under control is of paramount importance for overall health and wellness. Any excess ammonia generated by the CBS C699T+ mutation can drain stores of BH4. This will impact upon serotonin levels and to a certain extent cause fluxes in dopamine (which translates into mood swings). Therefore, keeping the CBS C699T+ mutation under control is of paramount importance to getting the body back in balance. Also helping to restore adequate levels of BH4 should aid in serotonin synthesis, maintaining dopamine levels in a more stable manner as well as ammonia detoxification.

In order to address the CBS C699T, it has been found that the use of a low protein diet, in conjunction with ammonia support RNA (1/2 dropper given with methylation cycle supplements and with every meal) will help to balance the system. It will make a big difference if protein in the diet is limited to those foods that will help to support healthy neurotransmitter levels. As discussed above, the balance of high tyrosine and high tryptophan foods should be decided based upon the COMT and VDR Bsm/Taq status. In addition the nightly use of charcoal as a supplement just before bed has proven to aid in controlling excess ammonia levels. In addition the nightly use of charcoal as a supplement just before bed has proven to aid in controlling excess ammonia levels. The use of charcoal just prior to bed should separate the time frame of the addition of the charcoal from other supporting supplements. This should limit the ability to of the charcoal to deplete the body of needed nutrients. It is important to be sure that the bowels are moving well with the addition of charcoal. The use of a magnesium citrate flush (high doses of magnesium citrate) following the addition of 1 to 2 charcoal capsules helps to ensure a bowel movement after this addition of charcoal to soak up excess ammonia. In addition the herb Yucca is reported to aid in ammonia support. The suggested starting dosage is ½ Yucca capsule per day.

A source of low dose P5P rather than a high dose B6 supplement is useful to support the body's B6 requiring reactions and at the same time, not acting to push the CBS reaction. The HHC Neurological Health general vitamin is a very good source of P5P and the other Bs for individuals with CBS C699T mutations in spite of the fact that it does have low concentrations of sulfur containing compounds. It is a bit of a "catch 22"; the body does need the sulfur compounds such as glutathione, but it creates more difficulties when they are added until the CBS mutation has been addressed from a nutritional standpoint. These supplements should help to deal with both aspects of this issue.

The CBS C699T mutation will not only deplete the intermediates in the methylation cycle, it will also lead to elevated levels of taurine and excess sulfur groups. It is recommend that individuals with a CBS C699T+ mutation do not use high levels of taurine or additional sulfur donors (broccoli etc) as it may create problems with excess sulfur groups (a small amount in a general vitamin is okay but using 500mg taurine capsules is not recommended).

The CBS C699T mutation will also cause a depletion of molybdenum levels as molybdenum is involved in making sulfur groups less toxic in the body as it is a cofactor for the enzyme sulfite oxidase. Increased amounts of molybdenum may be utilized in individuals with a CBS C699T up regulation in response to the increased generation of sulfur groups via the transulfuration reaction. It may be hard to keep molybdenum in the normal range and this may account in part for copper/ zinc imbalances that are observed as the molybdenum cannot keep up. It is worth running an essential mineral urine test to be certain that molybdenum levels are in the normal range. If not, it would make sense to consider using molybdenum supplementation; the E lyte molybdenum is an easily absorbed source of this mineral. On a related note, xanthine oxidase is another molybdenum requiring enzyme in the body. When milk and other dairy products are not homogenized, components of the milk are digested in the stomach and the small intestine, including the enzyme xanthine oxidase. However, when milk is homogenized, its xanthine oxidase is not broken down but instead passes into the general circulation of the body. The elevated presence of xanthine oxidase may exacerbate limited molybdenum levels and add to further imbalances in the copper levels. This would also suggest that it is wise to continue with a casein free diet and that if you are going to use any dairy products that it may be beneficial to use whole dairy products that are not homogenized particularly for individuals with CBS C699T mutations. Molybdenum, EDTA, carnosine and zinc will help to keep copper/zinc ratios in a more appropriate balance. Chewable zinc tablets with slippery elm will benefit the gut as well as providing a well controlled dose of zinc. Dosing can start with ¼ tablet and increase to 1 whole tablet per day. The E lyte zinc is an acceptable alternative. BioNativius trace minerals are useful for providing general mineral support along with additional support as needed from the E lyte zinc, molybdenum and magnesium. Essential mineral tests can be run from urine samples to verify that minerals are within range. Pay careful attention to lithium and iodine levels during any detoxification of heavy metals as excretion of mercury can affect the levels of lithium and iodine. These essential minerals appear to play an important role in helping to balance mood swings that can occur as a result of dopamine fluxes. These dopamine fluxes are much more of an issue in individuals who are COMT + +   regardless of their VDR Bsm and Taq status. If lithium of lithium or iodine levels are low, useful supplements to support healthy levels include lithium oratate and iodoral. A suggested starting dose is ¼ of each tablet/capsule daily.

As a further result of the CBS C699T+ mutation, there may be high taurine and very low levels of homocysteine on a urine amino acid test. Individuals with this mutation also tend to have more difficulties with sulfur containing compounds. This would include garlic, broccoli, taurine, glutathione, and even DMPS and DMSA. Once the body is supported nutritionally to address the CBS mutation these individuals are in a better position to be able to use sulfur containing compounds including glutathione.

The CBS C699T will also put some strain on the urea cycle. The availability of BH4 helps to determine whether nitric oxide, peroxy nitrite or super oxide is formed as a function of the urea cycle. Two molecules of BH4 are required for formation of nitric oxide; one molecule of BH4 leads to the formation of peroxy nitrite and the absence of BH4 leads to super oxide formation. The BH4 acts in concert with the NOS enzyme in the urea cycle to produce these end products. There is some literature to suggest that omega 3 EFAs may limit the activity of NOS. As with most other supplements this suggests that moderation is the best approach. The use of an EFA mixture that has omega 3:6:9 every other day, alternating it with source of omega 3 fatty acids such as DHA should help to strike a reasonable balance in individuals with NOS mutations. For those individuals who do not have NOS mutations, the daily use of an omega 3 mixture in addition to the daily use of a separate source of omega 3s should be fine. In this way the body is supported for optimal membrane fluidity, yet at the same time is limiting any negative effects of too much omega 3 on the NOS enzyme. A lower protein diet and the use of Stress RNA once or twice daily will also help to take some of the strain off of the urea cycle. A strain on the urea cycle due to inefficient NOS activity can lead to elevated levels of ammonia that can exacerbate the ammonia problem as a result of the CBS C699T+ mutations and lead to further drains on the already limited stores of BH4.

Preliminary collaborative research is ongoing between myself and a group of doctors in Japan, looking at the use of prescription BH4 to help to compensate for MTHFR A1298C and CBS C699T+ mutations. The initial results in this area are encouraging. Low daily doses of BH4 initially appear to stimulate detoxification over the first several weeks of use. After this initial detoxification effect the BH4 appears to have a very positive impact on language for individuals with CBS C699T+ mutations.

In addition to addressing the CBS C699T mutation, it is important to supplement the methylation pathway to ensure that there are adequate methyl and sulfur donors for the body.

Once the CBS up regulation has been addressed, individuals are in a better position to maintain appropriate levels of intermediates in the pathway once they have been added to his/her system, rather than having them drain through the CBS C699T which as currently acting like a "hole in the bucket".

- CBS C699T + or + +
- MTR - -
- MTRR - -

We are fortunate in that he/she does not have mutations in the methionine synthase or the methionine synthase reductase genes. This would suggest that that he/she should not be severely depleted in methyl B12 once the CBS C699T + mutation is adequately addressed so that is not draining his/her methylation cycle intermediates from his/her system. As part of a comprehensive program it would still be wise to supplement with some B12; however, high levels of supplementation should not be necessary as he/she does not have mutations in this specific aspect of the pathway. Individuals who are COMT + + should use hydroxy B12 for supplementation where as those who are more limited in methyl groups due to their COMT VDR status should use methyl B12.

There is a second pathway to the formation of methionine through the BHMT enzyme that will bypass mutations in the methionine synthase and methionine synthase reductase genes. Again, as with the supplementation with B12, it is advisable to support these pathways. However high level supplementation should not be necessary as there are no mutations that have been noted on the nutrigenomic test in the ability to utilize and regenerate methyl B12. This pathway uses phosphatidyl serine and /or TMG as donors for the reaction. It is wise to consider adding PS and a small amount of TMG to help to drive this reaction. While DMG works well to support language, it may be best to wait to add any DMG until this pathway is supplemented properly, as the DMG may be inhibiting this BHMT reaction to methionine. Supplementation for this part of the pathway also uses a low dose of TMG, choline and plain methionine. The HHC general vitamin is acceptable as a source for TMG, choline and methionine as well as the other general nutrients contained in it (½-1 in the morning and another ½-1 in the afternoon). In addition, phosphatidyl serine should also be added to help to support the "back door" reaction from homocysteine to methionine via the BHMT enzyme. Phosphatidyl serine is available as plain PS gel caps as well as a chewable form with DMAE (Pedi-Active). DMAE contains methyl groups so this is an ideal form for individuals who need extra methyl groups based on their COMT and VDR test results. Plain phosphatidyl serine is often available as a gelcap and this is a preferred form. Individuals who are COMT ++ should use only the plain phosphatidyl serine gel caps. Those in need of additional methyl groups due to their COMT and VDR status should consider using one phosphatidyl serine gel cap as well as one of the chewable Pedi-Active PS with DMAE daily.

COMT + + individuals should also be supporting the rest of the methylation pathway with ¼ Intrinsic B12, ¼ nucleotides, ¼ dropper methylation support RNA, as well as appropriate support for the CBS up regulation and for the BHMT reaction described above.

COMT - - individuals should also be supporting the rest of the methylation pathway with ¼ Folapro, ¼ Intrinsic B12, ¼ nucleotides, ¼ dropper methylation support RNA, as well as appropriate support for the CBS upregulation and for the BHMT reaction described above.

CBS - -
(no upregulation)

- ## CBS C699T - - (no upregulation)

There is no CBS C699T mutation and he/she also does not have a NOS mutation. While you do not need to use an excessively low protein diet, you should be cognizant of the amount of protein that you are using in the diet and consider using Stress RNA to help to take any strain off of the urea cycle due to ingestion of proteins. A lower protein diet and the use of Stress RNA once or twice daily will also help to take some of the strain off of the urea cycle; you can consider using the Stress RNA once or twice daily. There is some literature to suggest that omega 3 EFAs may limit the activity of NOS. As with most other supplements this suggests that moderation is the best approach. The use of an EFA mixture that has omega 3:6:9 every day, along with a source of omega 3 fatty acids such as DHA should help to strike a reasonable balance in individuals with no NOS mutations. In this way the body is supported for optimal membrane fluidity, yet at the same time is limiting any negative effects of too much omega 3 on the NOS enzyme. A strain on the urea cycle due to inefficient NOS activity or high protein levels can lead to elevated levels of ammonia that are sufficient to cause flapping and other over stimulatory behaviors. If you are finding high ammonia levels upon testing you can consider the weekly use of charcoal as a supplement (many individuals find it convenient to do the charcoal protocol on a weekend). The nightly use of charcoal as a supplement just before bed has proven to aid in controlling excess ammonia levels. The use of charcoal just prior to bed should separate the time frame of the addition of the charcoal from other supporting supplements. This should limit the ability to of the charcoal to deplete the body of needed nutrients. It is important to be sure that the bowels are moving well with the addition of charcoal. The use of a magnesium citrate flush (high doses of magnesium citrate) following the addition of 1 to 2 charcoal capsules helps to ensure a bowel movement after this addition of charcoal to soak up excess ammonia. In addition, the herb Yucca is reported to aid in ammonia support. The suggested starting dosage is ½ Yucca capsule per day.

Where this nutrigenomic test does not show a CBS C699T mutation or an NOS mutation which can lead to elevated ammonia levels, it does not rule out other imbalances that can cause increased ammonia. Since I am not certain of the diet that you are following, I will address the use of the diet in general, as it relates to the genetics at this time. I do understand that the SCD diet has made a big difference for a number of individuals and this diet is acceptable for individuals like you who do not have mutations in CBS C699T or NOS mutations. However, if you are supplementing protein it is important to monitor ammonia levels to be certain that the body is able to dispose of the ammonia properly which is generated from the intake of high protein foods. The SCD diet appears to benefit a number of individuals with prior gut issues Excess stomach acid in the system can cause loose stools and severe stomach pain that is often seen in these individuals. Ammonia that is generated from excessive protein is alkaline. This can help to neutralize the stomach acid and can help to make the stools firmer and gut pain better. However, by neutralizing the stomach acid, it does not deal directly with the root of the problem, if it is caused by excess stomach acid. Stomach acid can be triggered by histamine reacting with H2 receptors in the stomach. So, a high protein diet may be increasing ammonia which is neutralizing the stomach acid and improving the gut issue. However, it is not addressing the source of any excess acid or high histamine in the system and other consequences of high ammonia. The body uses two molecules of BH4 to detoxify one molecule of ammonia to urea. This is an expensive way to use our BH4. BH4 is also needed for dopamine and serotonin as well as language related function. Since language is a primary problem for many children, using up limited BH4 to detoxify ammonia may not be the best use of it for the body. I am not suggesting that parents abandon the SCD diet, especially as it has made a positive difference for many children. What is suggested is that you run a DDI urine amino acid test so that you can look at ammonia levels and amino acids while the child is on the SCD diet. Arginine and citrulline imbalances may indicate problems in other aspects of ammonia detoxification that can also lead to elevated ammonia. For individuals who are CBS C699T negative, yet still have elevated ammonia levels, it would be worth considering additional nutrigenomic testing to rule out OTC mutations in the urea cycle if they are not using a high protein diet. I would also suggest a test for helicobacter as that is often a causative agent for excess stomach acid. The use of mastica gum is very helpful for addressing this organism; the suggested dosage is ½ mastica gum, Stomach pH and Bowel Support with meals.

- CBS - - NOS + or +

Although there is no CBS C699T mutation, he/she does have a NOS mutation. While you do not need to use an excessively low protein diet, a lower protein diet and the use of Stress RNA will help to take some of the strain off of the urea cycle due to the NOS mutation. You should consider using the Stress RNA once or twice daily. There is some literature to suggest that omega 3 EFAs may limit the activity of NOS. As with most other supplements this suggests that moderation is the best approach. The use of an EFA mixture that has omega 3:6:9 every other day, alternating it with a source of omega 3 fatty acids such as DHA should help to strike a reasonable balance in individuals with NOS mutations. For those individuals who do not have NOS mutations, the daily use of an omega 3 mixture in addition to the daily use of a separate source of omega 3s should be fine. In this way the body is supported for optimal membrane fluidity, yet at the same time is limiting any negative effects of too much omega 3 on the NOS enzyme. A lower protein diet and the use of Stress RNA once or twice daily will also help to take some of the strain off of the urea cycle. A strain on the urea cycle due to inefficient NOS activity can lead to elevated levels of ammonia that are sufficient to cause flapping and other over stimulatory behaviors. As a consequence, in addition to a lower protein diet you should consider the weekly use of charcoal as a supplement (many individuals find it convenient to do the charcoal protocol on a weekend). The nightly use of charcoal as a supplement just before bed has proven to aid in controlling excess ammonia levels. The use of charcoal just prior to bed should separate the time frame of the addition of the charcoal from other supporting supplements. This should limit the ability to of the charcoal to deplete the body of needed nutrients. It is important to be sure that the bowels are moving well with the addition of charcoal. The use of a magnesium citrate flush (high doses of magnesium citrate) following the addition of 1 to 2 charcoal capsules helps to ensure a bowel movement after this addition of charcoal to soak up excess ammonia. In addition the herb Yucca is reported to aid in ammonia support. The suggested starting dosage is ½ Yucca capsule per day.

Again, where this test does not show a CBS C699T mutation which can lead to elevated ammonia levels it does not rule out other imbalances that can cause increased ammonia. For individuals who are CBS C699T negative, yet still have elevated ammonia levels, it would be worth considering additional nutrigenomic testing to rule out OTC mutations in the urea cycle. You can also run a DDI urine amino acid test so that you can look at ammonia levels and amino acids; arginine (high) and citrulline (low) imbalances may indicate problems in other aspects of the ammonia detoxification that can also lead to elevated ammonia levels.

Mitochondrial Support

- Mitochondrial Support
- COMT + +
- VDR Bsm/Taq + + or VDR Bsm/Taq + - or VDR Bsm/Taq - -

To aid in the detoxification process as well as to support mitochondrial energy it is beneficial to use a mitochondrial support cocktail. This cocktail consists of carnitine, ATP, CoQ10, Idebenone and NADH. (Decreased mitochondrial energy can lead to fatigue, low muscle tone, muscle weakness as well as fine and gross motor issues.) ATP and NADH can be used on a daily basis.

Carnitine, CoQ10 and Idebenone all contain methyl groups. Where he/she is COMT + + it is best to rotate these methyl containing supplements rather than using them on a daily basis. For this reason it is also advisable to use only 50mg for the c of CoQ10, Idebenone and carnitine. CoQ10 (50mg) can be used on day one, Idebenone on day two, carnitine on day three, and then repeat this pattern on day four. You may want to start by using only ½ of each of these supplements and then gradually increasing the dosages. By supporting the mitochondria with these supplements it should help to aid in energy production and the detoxification process. The mitochondrial cocktail can be added after the methylation support so that you are not adding too many supplements that stimulate detoxification at the same time.

In addition to its role in mitochondrial support, increased levels of NAD have also been shown to slow degeneration of axons in animal models of neurodegenerative disease and peripheral neuropathies. NAD levels were found to decrease in degenerating axons and increasing the level of NAD and/or nicotinamide was able to offer protection. NADH is also helpful for chronic bacterial infection and also for individuals

with glucose 6 phosphate dehydrogenase deficiencies. A separate nutrigenomic test panel is available to evaluate glucose 6 phosphate dehydrogenase mutations. The panel looks at 100 different SNPs or variants for G6PDH; obviously this is a common genetic mutation with fairly widespread distribution in the population. A deficiency of this enzyme creates problems with recycling glutathione. The use of NADH will help to reduce any oxidized glutathione and so the use of NADH may be useful in part to compensate for decreased G6PDH activity. On the other hand sulfur donors can decrease the activity of this enzyme, even if there is no mutation present. This fact is known and characterized. If you have one of the many mutations that lead to decreased activity of this enzyme then sulfur excess will be more of an issue. Deficiencies in the G6PDH enzyme cause the RBCs to be more fragile and to rupture easily leading to anemia. A G6PDH deficiency could create issues with sulfur donors and may cause problems with the use of DHEA or sulfur based chelating agents in any form including transdermal forms; potential symptoms of a sulfur toxicity problem can include broken capillaries, excessive bruising and bleeding, nose bleeds and problems with sugar regulation as well as decreased levels of 5 carbon sugars in the body. Where RBCs have a half life of 120 days in the body, it can take several months for the excess sulfur to build to a point where they have a cumulative effect on the G6PDH levels in the RBCs. It is especially important for individuals using sulfur based products to watch for signs of sulfur toxicity that manifest over the course of several months, such as broken capillaries, increased bruising, or decreased kidney function. If you do see any of these symptoms you may want to consider taking a break from the use of sulfur based products. The addition of NADH should be helpful for potential problems with G6PDH. When the G6PDH enzyme is not functioning properly, it will lead to higher levels of free glucose which can lead to bursts of insulin. This can in turn create further inflammation in the body. The use of thyroid supplementation and adrenal supplementation, alternative sources of 5 carbon sugars such as Ambrotose and the Beyond C form of vitamin C with ribose should also help to support decreased levels of G6PDH.

By supporting the mitochondria with NADH, as well as the rest of the mitochondrial cocktail it should help the body to have the necessary energy for detoxification and also may help to compensate for any mutations or deletions in SOD or in the glutathione pathway.

It may also be worth considering nutritional support for the Krebs cycle in the body. The Krebs cycle (also known as the TCA cycle) is responsible for helping to generate energy via reactions that take place in the mitochondria. The Krebs cycle is tied to our complete methylation cycle diagram via fumarate and aspartate that are part of the urea cycle. Fumarate and aspartate also a key intermediates of the Krebs cycle. Low levels of fumarate as a result of excess ammonia, OTC mutations, or NOS mutations may have a negative impact on the Krebs cycle. It possible to supplement the Krebs cycle directly with carnitine fumarate to help to compensate for low fumarate due to urea cycle issues. It is also worth considering additional Krebs cycle support based on the levels of Krebs cycle intermediates on an organic acid test. As already mentioned, it is possible to supplement with fumarate individually as well as to use forms of vitamin E succinate as a means to supplement low levels of succinate. The conversion of methylmalonyl Co A to succinyl CoA requires B12.

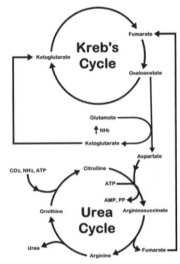

Individuals with mutations in MTR and MTRR may show low levels of succinate due to decreased levels of B12. In addition to supporting for the MTR and MTRR mutations, it may be useful to also supplement directly with Vitamin E succinate to take some of the strain off of the need to B12 and to support the Krebs cycle directly with this intermediate. Malic acid is often used to chelate aluminum; however it will also support healthy levels of malate in the Krebs cycle. Magnesium citrate can serve as a source of magnesium supplementation as well as a source of citrate for the Kreb's cycle.

More general overall Krebs cycle support can include nutrients such as pyruvate or methyl pyruvate (not for COMT++) and supplements entitled "Krebs cycle intermediates" (provided they do not include glutamate, aspartate or their derivatives), such as zinc in a complex with Krebs cycle intermediates. Again, testing to determine the level of various Krebs cycle intermediates should be done before deciding on which supplements to utilize.

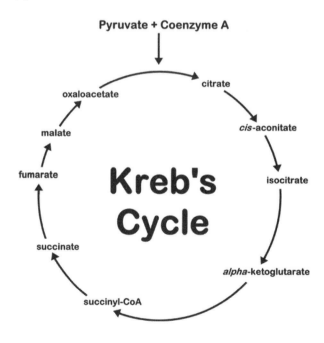

- Mitochondrial Support
- COMT - -
- VDR Bsm/Taq - -

To aid in the detoxification process as well as to support mitochondrial energy it is beneficial to use a mitochondrial support cocktail. This cocktail consists of carnitine, ATP, CoQ10, Idebenone and NADH. (Decreased mitochondrial energy can lead to fatigue, low muscle tone, muscle weakness as well as fine and gross motor issues.) ATP and NADH can be used on a daily basis.

Carnitine, CoQ10 and Idebenone all contain methyl groups. Where he/she is COMT --/VDR - -it is best to rotate these methyl containing supplements rather than using them on a daily basis. For this reason it is also advisable to use only 50mg for the CoQ10 and alternate the use of CoQ10, Idebenone and carnitine. CoQ10 (50mg) can be used on day one, Idebenone on day two, carnitine on day three, and then repeat this pattern on day four. You may want to start by using only ½ of each of these supplements and then gradually increasing the dosages. By supporting the mitochondria with these supplements it should help to aid in energy production and the detoxification process. The mitochondrial cocktail can be added after the methylation support so that you are not adding too many supplements that stimulate detoxification at the same time.

In addition to its role in mitochondrial support, increased levels of NAD have also been shown to slow degeneration of axons in animal models of neurodegenerative disease and peripheral neuropathies. NAD levels were found to decrease in degenerating axons and increasing the level of NAD and/or nicotinamide was able to offer protection. NADH is also helpful for chronic bacterial infection and also for individuals

with glucose 6 phosphate dehydrogenase deficiencies. A separate nutrigenomic test panel is available to evaluate Glucose 6 phosphate dehydrogenase mutations. The panel looks at 100 different SNPs or variants for G6PDH; obviously this is a common genetic mutation with fairly widespread distribution in the population. A deficiency of this enzyme creates problems with recycling glutathione. The use of NADH will help to reduce any oxidized glutathione and so the use of NADH may be useful in part to compensate for decreased G6PDH activity. On the other hand sulfur donors can decrease the activity of this enzyme, even if there is no mutation present. This fact is known and characterized. If you have one of the many mutations that lead to decreased activity of this enzyme then sulfur excess will be more of an issue. Deficiencies in the G6PDH enzyme cause the RBCs to be more fragile and to rupture easily leading to anemia. A G6PDH deficiency could create issues with sulfur donors and may cause problems with the use of DHEA or sulfur based chelating agents in any form including transdermal forms; potential symptoms of a sulfur toxicity problem can include broken capillaries, excessive bruising and bleeding, nose bleeds and problems with sugar regulation as well as decreased levels of 5 carbon sugars in the body. Where RBCs have a half life of 120 days in the body, it can take several months for the excess sulfur to build to a point where they have a cumulative effect on the G6PDH levels in the RBCs. It is especially important for individuals using sulfur based products to watch for signs of sulfur toxicity that manifest over the course of several months, such as broken capillaries, increased bruising, or decreased kidney function. If you do see any of these symptoms you may want to consider taking a break from the use of sulfur based products. The addition of NADH should be helpful for potential problems with G6PDH. When the G6PDH enzyme is not functioning properly, it will lead to higher levels of free glucose which can lead to bursts of insulin. This can in turn create further inflammation in the body. The use of thyroid supplementation and adrenal supplementation, alternative sources of 5 carbon sugars such as Ambrotose and the Beyond C form of vitamin C with ribose should also help to support decreased levels of G6PDH.

By supporting the mitochondria with NADH, as well as the rest of the mitochondrial cocktail it should help the body to have the necessary energy for detoxification and also may help to compensate for any mutations or deletions in SOD or in the glutathione pathway.

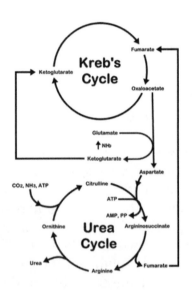

It may also be worth considering nutritional support for the Krebs cycle in the body. The Krebs cycle (also known as the TCA cycle) is responsible for helping to generate energy via reactions that take place in the mitochondria. The Krebs cycle is tied to our complete methylation cycle diagram via fumarate and aspartate that are part of the urea cycle. Fumarate and aspartate also a key intermediates of the Krebs cycle. Low levels of fumarate as a result of excess ammonia, OTC mutations, or NOS mutations may have a negative impact on the Krebs cycle. It possible to supplement the Krebs cycle directly with carnitine fumarate to help to compensate for low fumarate due to urea cycle issues. It is also worth considering additional Krebs cycle support based on the levels of Krebs cycle intermediates on an organic acid test. As already mentioned, it is possible to supplement with fumarate individually as well as to use forms of vitamin E succinate as a means to supplement low levels of succinate. The conversion of methylmalonyl Co A to succinyl CoA requires B12. Individuals with mutations in MTR and MTRR may show low levels of succinate due to decreased levels of B12. In addition to supporting for the MTR and MTRR mutations, it may be useful to also supplement directly with Vitamin E succinate to take some of the strain off of the need to B12 and to support the Krebs cycle directly with this intermediate. Malic acid is often used to chelate aluminum; however it will also support healthy levels of malate in the Krebs cycle. Magnesium citrate can serve as a source of magnesium supplementation as well as a source of citrate for the Kreb's cycle.

More general overall Krebs cycle support can include nutrients such as pyruvate or methyl pyruvate (not for COMT++) and supplements entitled "Krebs cycle intermediates" (provided they do not include glutamate, aspartate or their derivatives), such as zinc in a complex with Krebs cycle intermediates. Again, testing to determine the level of various Krebs cycle intermediates should be done before deciding on which supplements to utilize.

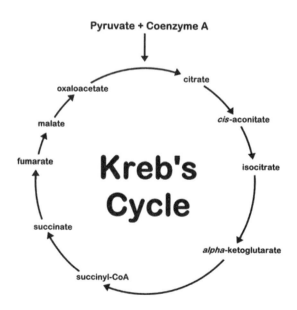

- Mitochondrial Support
- COMT - -
- VDR Bsm/Taq + + or VDR Bsm/Taq + -

To aid in the detoxification process as well as to support mitochondrial energy it is beneficial to use a mitochondrial support cocktail. This cocktail consists of carnitine, ATP, CoQ10, Idebenone and NADH. (Decreased mitochondrial energy can lead to fatigue, low muscle tone, muscle weakness as well as fine and gross motor issues.) ATP and NADH can be used on a daily basis.

Carnitine, CoQ10 and Idebenone all contain methyl groups and as he/she is COMT - - his/her system may be depleted in these groups and should require daily supplementation with carnitine, CoQ10 and Idebenone. He/she should be able to tolerate one of each of these supplements. In addition, he/she should be able to handle a higher dose of CoQ10, 200mg. per day. If there is any problem in tolerating one whole capsule of each then start with only ½ of each of these supplements and then gradually increasing the dosages. By supporting the mitochondria with these supplements it should help to aid in energy production and the detoxification process. The mitochondrial cocktail can be added after the methylation support so that you are not adding too many supplements that stimulate detoxification at the same time.

In addition to its role in mitochondrial support, increased levels of NAD have also been shown to slow degeneration of axons in animal models of neurodegenerative disease and peripheral neuropathies. NAD levels were found to decrease in degenerating axons and increasing the level of NAD and/or nicotinamide was able to offer protection. NADH is also helpful for chronic bacterial infection and also for individuals with glucose 6 phosphate dehydrogenase deficiencies. A separate nutrigenomic test panel is available to evaluate Glucose 6 phosphate dehydrogenase mutations. The panel looks at 100 different SNPs or variants for G6PDH; obviously this is a common genetic mutation with fairly widespread distribution in the population. A deficiency of this enzyme creates problems with recycling glutathione. The use of NADH will help to reduce any oxidized glutathione and so the use of NADH may be useful in part to compensate for decreased G6PDH activity. On the other hand sulfur donors can decrease the activity of this enzyme, even if there is no mutation present. This fact is known and characterized. If you have one of the many mutations that lead to decreased activity of this enzyme then sulfur excess will be more of an issue. This problem will be compounded by excess sulfur groups that are generated by the CBS up regulation (the CBS C699T mutation). Regardless of the G6PDH mutation status, the use of high dose sulfur donors (such as those generated by the CBS C699T+) can create a deficiency of this enzyme over time. Deficiencies in the G6PDH enzyme cause the RBCs to be more fragile and to rupture easily leading to anemia. If he/she does have a G6PDH deficiency in addition to his/her CBS C699T+ status it would create issues with sulfur donors and may cause problems with the use of DHEA or sulfur based chelating agents in any form including transdermal forms; potential symptoms of a sulfur toxicity problem can include broken capillaries, excessive bruising and bleeding, nose bleeds and problems with sugar regulation as well as decreased levels of 5 carbon sugars in the body. Where RBCs have a half life of 120 days in the body, it can take several months for the excess sulfur to build to a point where they have a cumulative effect on the G6PDH levels in the RBCs. It is especially important for individuals with CBS C699T mutations who are using sulfur based products to watch for signs of sulfur toxicity that manifest over the course of several months, such as broken capillaries, increased bruising, or decreased kidney function. If you do see any of these symptoms you may want to consider taking a break from the use of sulfur based products. This is another reason that individuals with CBS C699T mutations should support the body with nutrients to address this issue and also try to limit the total number of sulfur donors in their system. The addition of NADH should be helpful for potential problems with G6PDH. When the G6PDH enzyme is not functioning properly, it will lead to higher levels of free glucose which can lead to bursts of insulin. This can in turn create further inflammation in the body. The use of thyroid supplementation and adrenal supplementation, alternative sources of 5 carbon sugars such as Ambrotose and the Beyond C form of vitamin C with ribose should also help to support decreased levels of G6PDH.

By supporting the mitochondria with NADH, as well as the rest of the mitochondrial cocktail it should help the body to have the necessary energy for detoxification and also may help to compensate for any mutations or deletions in SOD or in the glutathione pathway.

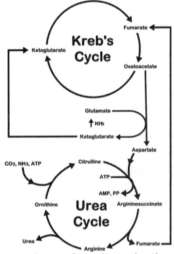

It may also be worth considering nutritional support for the Krebs cycle in the body. The Krebs cycle (also known as the TCA cycle) is responsible for helping to generate energy via reactions that take place in the mitochondria. The Krebs cycle is tied to our complete methylation cycle diagram via fumarate and aspartate that are part of the urea cycle. Fumarate and aspartate also a key intermediates of the Krebs cycle. Low levels of fumarate as a result of excess ammonia, OTC mutations, or NOS mutations may have a negative impact on the Krebs cycle. It possible to supplement the Krebs cycle directly with carnitine fumarate to help to compensate for low fumarate due to urea cycle issues. It is also worth considering additional Krebs cycle support based on the levels of Krebs cycle intermediates on an organic acid test. As already mentioned, it is possible to supplement with fumarate individually as well as to use forms of vitamin E succinate as a means to supplement low levels of succinate. The conversion of methylmalonyl Co A to succinyl CoA requires B12. Individuals with mutations in MTR and MTRR may show low levels of succinate due to decreased levels of B12. In addition to supporting for the MTR and MTRR mutations, it may be useful to also supplement directly with Vitamin E succinate to take some of the strain off of the need to B12 and to support the Krebs cycle directly with this intermediate. Malic acid is often used to chelate aluminum; however it will also support healthy levels of malate in the Krebs cycle. Magnesium citrate can serve as a source of magnesium supplementation as well as a source of citrate for the Kreb's cycle.

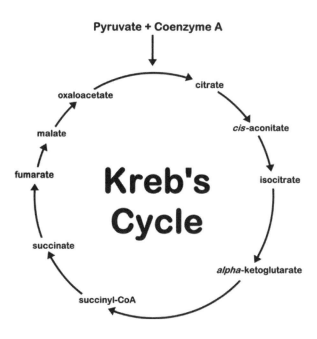

More general overall Krebs cycle support can include nutrients such as pyruvate or methyl pyruvate (not for COMT++) and supplements entitled "Krebs cycle intermediates" (provided they do not include glutamate, aspartate or their derivatives), such as zinc in a complex with Krebs cycle intermediates. Again, testing to determine the level of various Krebs cycle intermediates should be done before deciding on which supplements to utilize.

- Mitochondrial Support
- COMT + -
- VDR Bsm/Taq + +

To aid in the detoxification process as well as to support mitochondrial energy it is beneficial to use a mitochondrial support cocktail. This cocktail consists of carnitine, ATP, CoQ10, Idebenone and NADH. (Decreased mitochondrial energy can lead to fatigue, low muscle tone, muscle weakness as well as fine and gross motor issues.) ATP and NADH can be used on a daily basis.

Carnitine, CoQ10 and Idebenone all contain methyl groups. Where he/she is COMT + - it is best to rotate these methyl containing supplements rather than using them on a daily basis. For this reason it is also advisable to use 100mg of CoQ10 and alternate the use of CoQ10, Idebenone and carnitine. CoQ10 (100mg) can be used on day one, Idebenone on day two, carnitine on day three, and then repeat this pattern on day four. He/she should be able to tolerate one of each of these supplements. If there is any problem in tolerating one whole capsule of each then start with only ½ of each of these supplements and then gradually increasing the dosages. By supporting the mitochondria with these supplements it should help to aid in energy production and the detoxification process. The mitochondrial cocktail can be added after the methylation support so that you are not adding too many supplements that stimulate detoxification at the same time.

In addition to its role in mitochondrial support, increased levels of NAD have also been shown to slow degeneration of axons in animal models of neurodegenerative disease and peripheral neuropathies. NAD levels were found to decrease in degenerating axons and increasing the level of NAD and/or nicotinamide was able to offer protection. NADH is also helpful for chronic bacterial infection and also for individuals with glucose 6 phosphate dehydrogenase deficiencies. A separate nutrigenomic test panel is available to evaluate Glucose 6 phosphate dehydrogenase mutations. The panel looks at 100 different SNPs or variants for G6PDH; obviously this is a common genetic mutation with fairly widespread distribution in the population. A deficiency of this enzyme creates problems with recycling glutathione. The use of NADH will help to reduce any oxidized glutathione and so the use of NADH may be useful in part to compensate for decreased G6PDH activity. On the other hand sulfur donors can decrease the activity of this enzyme, even if there is no mutation present. This fact is known and characterized. If you have one of the many mutations that lead to decreased activity of this enzyme then sulfur excess will be more of an issue. This problem will be compounded by excess sulfur groups that are generated by the CBS up regulation (the CBS C699T mutation). Regardless of the G6PDH mutation status, the use of high dose sulfur donors (such as those generated by the CBS C699T+) can create a deficiency of this enzyme over time. Deficiencies in the G6PDH enzyme cause the RBCs to be more fragile and to rupture easily leading to anemia. If he/she does have a G6PDH deficiency in addition to his/her CBS C699T+ status it would create issues with sulfur donors and may cause problems with the use of DHEA or sulfur based chelating agents in any form including transdermal forms; potential symptoms of a sulfur toxicity problem can include broken capillaries, excessive bruising and bleeding, nose bleeds and problems with sugar regulation as well as decreased levels of 5 carbon sugars in the body. Where RBCs have a half life of 120 days in the body, it can take several months for the excess sulfur to build to a point where they have a cumulative effect on the G6PDH levels in the RBCs. It is especially important for individuals with CBS C699T mutations who are using sulfur based products to watch for signs of sulfur toxicity that manifest over the course of several months, such as broken capillaries, increased bruising, or decreased kidney function. Even without a CBS C699T mutation it is important to be cognizant of this issue. If you do see any of these symptoms you may want to consider taking a break from the use of sulfur based products. This is another reason that individuals with CBS C699T mutations should support the body with nutrients to address this issue and also try to limit the total number of sulfur donors in their system. The addition of NADH should be helpful for potential problems with G6PDH. When the G6PDH enzyme is not functioning properly, it will lead to higher levels of free glucose which can lead to bursts of insulin. This can in turn create further inflammation in the body. The use of thyroid supplementation and adrenal supplementation, alternative sources of 5 carbon sugars such as Ambrotose and the Beyond C form of vitamin C with ribose should also help to support decreased levels of G6PDH.

By supporting the mitochondria with NADH, as well as the rest of the mitochondrial cocktail it should help the body to have the necessary energy for detoxification and also may help to compensate for any mutations or deletions in SOD or in the glutathione pathway.

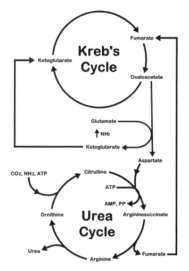

It may also be worth considering nutritional support for the Krebs cycle in the body. The Krebs cycle (also known as the TCA cycle) is responsible for helping to generate energy via reactions that take place in the mitochondria. The Krebs cycle is tied to our complete methylation cycle diagram via fumarate and aspartate that are part of the urea cycle. Fumarate and aspartate also a key intermediates of the Krebs cycle. Low levels of fumarate as a result of excess ammonia, OTC mutations, or NOS mutations may have a negative impact on the Krebs cycle. It possible to supplement the Krebs cycle directly with carnitine fumarate to help to compensate for low fumarate due to urea cycle issues. It is also worth considering additional Krebs cycle support based on the levels of Krebs cycle intermediates on an organic acid test. As already mentioned, it is possible to supplement with fumarate individually as well as to use forms of vitamin E succinate as a means to supplement low levels of succinate. The conversion of methylmalonyl Co A to succinyl CoA requires B12. Individuals with mutations in MTR and MTRR may show low levels of succinate due to decreased levels of B12. In addition to supporting for the MTR and MTRR mutations, it may be useful to also supplement directly with Vitamin E succinate to take some of the strain off of the need to B12 and to support the Krebs cycle directly with this intermediate. Malic acid is often used to chelate aluminum; however it will also support healthy levels of malate in the Krebs cycle. Magnesium citrate can serve as a source of

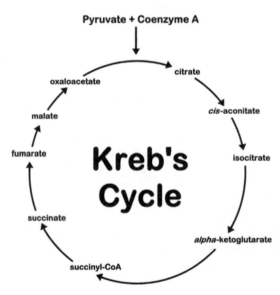

magnesium supplementation as well as a source of citrate for the Kreb's cycle.

More general overall Krebs cycle support can include nutrients such as pyruvate or methyl pyruvate (not for COMT++) and supplements entitled "Krebs cycle intermediates" (provided they do not include glutamate, aspartate or their derivatives), such as zinc in a complex with Krebs cycle intermediates. Again, testing to determine the level of various Krebs cycle intermediates should be done before deciding on which supplements to utilize.

- Mitochondrial Support
- COMT + -
- VDR Bsm/Taq - -

To aid in the detoxification process as well as to support mitochondrial energy it is beneficial to use a mitochondrial support cocktail. This cocktail consists of carnitine, ATP, CoQ10, Idebenone and NADH. (Decreased mitochondrial energy can lead to fatigue, low muscle tone, muscle weakness as well as fine and gross motor issues.) ATP and NADH can be used on a daily basis.

Carnitine, CoQ10 and Idebenone all contain methyl groups. Where he/she is COMT + + it is best to rotate these methyl containing supplements rather than using them on a daily basis. For this reason it is also advisable to use only 50mg for the CoQ10 and alternate the use of CoQ10, Idebenone and carnitine. CoQ10 (50mg) can be used on day one, Idebenone on day two, carnitine on day three, and then repeat this pattern on day four. You may want to start by using only ½ of each of these supplements and then gradually increasing the dosages. By supporting the mitochondria with these supplements it should help to aid in energy production and the detoxification process. The mitochondrial cocktail can be added after the methylation support so that you are not adding too many supplements that stimulate detoxification at the same time.

In addition to its role in mitochondrial support, increased levels of NAD have also been shown to slow degeneration of axons in animal models of neurodegenerative disease and peripheral neuropathies. NAD levels were found to decrease in degenerating axons and increasing the level of NAD and/or nicotinamide was able to offer protection. NADH is also helpful for chronic bacterial infection and also for individuals

with glucose 6 phosphate dehydrogenase deficiencies. A separate nutrigenomic test panel is available to evaluate Glucose 6 phosphate dehydrogenase mutations. The panel looks at 100 different SNPs or variants for G6PDH; obviously this is a common genetic mutation with fairly widespread distribution in the population. A deficiency of this enzyme creates problems with recycling glutathione. The use of NADH will help to reduce any oxidized glutathione and so the use of NADH may be useful in part to compensate for decreased G6PDH activity. On the other hand sulfur donors can decrease the activity of this enzyme even if there is no mutation present. This fact is known and characterized. If you have one of the many mutations that lead to decreased activity of this enzyme then sulfur excess will be more of an issue. This problem will be compounded by excess sulfur groups that are generated by the CBS up regulation (the CBS C699T mutation). Regardless of the G6PDH mutation status, the use of high dose sulfur donors (such as those generated by the CBS C699T+) can create a deficiency of this enzyme over time. Deficiencies in the G6PDH enzyme cause the RBCs to be more fragile and to rupture easily leading to anemia. If he/she does have a G6PDH deficiency in addition to his/her CBS C699T+ status it would create issues with sulfur donors and may cause problems with the use of DHEA or sulfur based chelating agents in any form including transdermal forms; potential symptoms of a sulfur toxicity problem can include broken capillaries, excessive bruising and bleeding, nose bleeds and problems with sugar regulation as well as decreased levels of 5 carbon sugars in the body. Where RBCs have a half life of 120 days in the body, it can take several months for the excess sulfur to build to a point where they have a cumulative effect on the G6PDH levels in the RBCs. It is especially important for individuals with CBS C699T mutations who are using sulfur based products to watch for signs of sulfur toxicity that manifest over the course of several months, such as broken capillaries, increased bruising, or decreased kidney function. If you do see any of these symptoms you may want to consider taking a break from the use of sulfur based products. This is another reason that individuals with CBS C699T mutations should support the body with nutrients to address this issue and also try to limit the total number of sulfur donors in their system. The addition of NADH should be helpful for potential problems with G6PDH. When the G6PDH enzyme is not functioning properly, it will lead to higher levels of free glucose which can lead to bursts of insulin. This can in turn create further inflammation in the body. The use of thyroid supplementation and adrenal supplementation, alternative sources of 5 carbon sugars such as Ambrotose and the Beyond C form of vitamin C with ribose should also help to support decreased levels of G6PDH.

By supporting the mitochondria with NADH as well as the rest of the mitochondrial cocktail it should help the body to have the necessary energy for detoxification and also may help to compensate for any mutations or deletions in SOD or in the glutathione pathway.

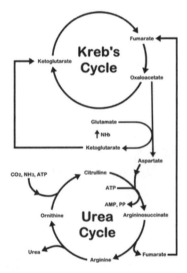

It may also be worth considering nutritional support for the Krebs cycle in the body. The Krebs cycle (also known as the TCA cycle) is responsible for helping to generate energy via reactions that take place in the mitochondria. The Krebs cycle is tied to our complete methylation cycle diagram via fumarate and aspartate that are part of the urea cycle. Fumarate and aspartate are also key intermediates of the Krebs cycle. Low levels of fumarate as a result of excess ammonia, OTC mutations, or NOS mutations may have a negative impact on the Krebs cycle. It is possible to supplement the Krebs cycle directly with carnitine fumarate to help to compensate for low fumarate due to urea cycle issues. It is also worth considering additional Krebs cycle support based on the levels of Krebs cycle intermediates on an organic acid test. As already mentioned, it is possible to supplement with fumarate individually as well as to use forms of vitamin E succinate as a means to supplement low levels of succinate. The conversion of methylmalonyl Co A to succinyl CoA requires B12. Individuals with mutations in MTR and MTRR may show low levels of succinate due to decreased levels of B12. In addition to supporting for the MTR and MTRR mutations, it may be useful to also supplement directly with Vitamin E succinate to take some of the strain off of the need for B12 and to support the Krebs cycle directly with this intermediate. Malic acid is often used to chelate aluminum; however it will also support healthy levels of malate in the Krebs cycle. Magnesium citrate can serve as a source of magnesium supplementation as well as a source of citrate for the Kreb's cycle.

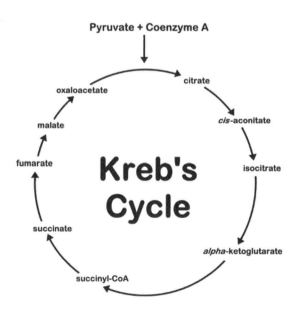

More general overall Krebs cycle support can include nutrients such as pyruvate or methyl pyruvate (not for COMT++) and supplements entitled "Krebs cycle intermediates" (provided they do not include glutamate, aspartate or their derivatives), such as zinc in a complex with Krebs cycle intermediates. Again, testing to determine the level of various Krebs cycle intermediates should be done before deciding on which supplements to utilize.

- Mitochondrial Support
- COMT + -
- VDR Bsm/Taq + -

To aid in the detoxification process as well as to support mitochondrial energy it is beneficial to use a mitochondrial support cocktail. This cocktail consists of carnitine, ATP, CoQ10, Idebenone and NADH. (Decreased mitochondrial energy can lead to fatigue, low muscle tone, muscle weakness as well as fine and gross motor issues.) ATP and NADH can be used on a daily basis.

Carnitine, CoQ10 and Idebenone all contain methyl groups. Where he/she is COMT + - it is best to rotate these methyl containing supplements rather than using them on a daily basis. For this reason it is also advisable to use 100mg of CoQ10 and alternate the use of CoQ10, Idebenone and carnitine. CoQ10 (100mg) can be used on day one, Idebenone on day two, carnitine on day three, and then repeat this pattern on day four. He/she should be able to tolerate one of each of these supplements. If there is any problem in tolerating one whole capsule of each then start with only ½ of each of these supplements and then gradually increasing the dosages. By supporting the mitochondria with these supplements it should help to aid in energy production and the detoxification process. The mitochondrial cocktail can be added after the methylation support so that you are not adding too many supplements that stimulate detoxification at the same time.

In addition to its role in mitochondrial support, increased levels of NAD have also been shown to slow degeneration of axons in animal models of neurodegenerative disease and peripheral neuropathies. NAD levels were found to decrease in degenerating axons and increasing the level of NAD and/or nicotinamide was able to offer protection. NADH is also helpful for chronic bacterial infection and also for individuals with glucose 6 phosphate dehydrogenase deficiencies. A separate nutrigenomic test panel is available to evaluate glucose 6 phosphate dehydrogenase mutations. The panel looks at 100 different SNPs or variants for G6PDH; obviously this is a common genetic mutation with fairly widespread distribution in the population. A deficiency of this enzyme creates problems with recycling glutathione. The use of NADH will help to reduce any oxidized glutathione and so the use of NADH may be useful in part to compensate for decreased G6PDH activity. On the other hand sulfur donors can decrease the activity of this enzyme even if there is no mutation present. This fact is known and characterized. If you have one of the many mutations that lead to decreased activity of this enzyme then sulfur excess will be more of an issue. This problem will be compounded by excess sulfur groups that are generated by the CBS up regulation (the CBS C699T mutation). Regardless of the G6PDH mutation status, the use of high dose sulfur donors (such as those generated by the CBS C699T+) can create a deficiency of this enzyme over time. Deficiencies in the G6PDH enzyme cause the RBCs to be more fragile and to rupture easily leading to anemia. If he/she does have a G6PDH deficiency in addition to his/her CBS C699T+ status it would create issues with sulfur donors and may cause problems with the use of DHEA or sulfur based chelating agents in any form including transdermal forms; potential symptoms of a sulfur toxicity problem can include broken capillaries, excessive bruising and bleeding, nose bleeds and problems with sugar regulation as well as decreased levels of 5 carbon sugars in the body. Where RBCs have a half life of 120 days in the body, it can take several months for the excess sulfur to build to a point where they have a cumulative effect on the G6PDH levels in the RBCs. It is especially important for individuals with CBS C699T mutations who are using sulfur based products to watch for signs of sulfur toxicity that manifest over the course of several months, such as broken capillaries, increased bruising, or decreased kidney function. Even without a CBS C699T mutation it is important to be cognizant of this issue. If you do see any of these symptoms you may want to consider taking a break from the use of sulfur based products. This is another reason that individuals with CBS C699T mutations should support the body with nutrients to address this issue and also try to limit the total number of sulfur donors in their system. The addition of NADH should be helpful for potential problems with G6PDH. When the G6PDH enzyme is not functioning properly, it will lead to higher levels of free glucose which can lead to bursts of insulin. This can in turn create further inflammation in the body. The use of thyroid supplementation and adrenal supplementation, alternative sources of 5 carbon sugars such as Ambrotose and the Beyond C form of vitamin C with ribose should also help to support decreased levels of G6PDH.

By supporting the mitochondria with NADH as well as the rest of the mitochondrial cocktail it should help the body to have the necessary energy for detoxification and also may help to compensate for any mutations or deletions in SOD or in the glutathione pathway.

It may also be worth considering nutritional support for the Krebs cycle in the body. The Krebs cycle (also known as the TCA cycle) is responsible for helping to generate energy via reactions that take place in the mitochondria. The Krebs cycle is tied to our complete methylation cycle diagram via fumarate and

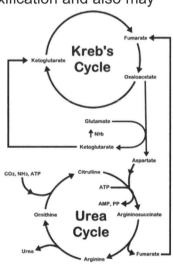

aspartate that are part of the urea cycle. Fumarate and aspartate are also key intermediates of the Krebs cycle. Low levels of fumarate as a result of excess ammonia, OTC mutations, or NOS mutations may have a negative impact on the Krebs cycle. It is possible to supplement the Krebs cycle directly with carnitine fumarate to help to compensate for low fumarate due to urea cycle issues. It is also worth considering additional Krebs cycle support based on the levels of Krebs cycle intermediates on an organic acid test. As already mentioned, it is possible to supplement with fumarate individually as well as to use forms of vitamin E succinate as a means to supplement low levels of succinate. The conversion of methylmalonyl Co A to succinyl CoA requires B12. Individuals with mutations in MTR and MTRR may show low levels of succinate due to decreased levels of B12. In addition to supporting for the MTR and MTRR mutations, it may be useful to also supplement directly with Vitamin E succinate to take some of the strain off of the need for B12 and to support

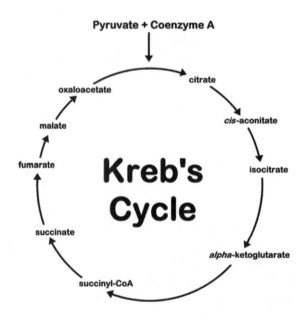

the Krebs cycle directly with this intermediate. Malic acid is often used to chelate aluminum; however it will also support healthy levels of malate in the Krebs cycle. Magnesium citrate can serve as a source of magnesium supplementation as well as a source of citrate for the Kreb's cycle.

More general overall Krebs cycle support can include nutrients such as pyruvate or methyl pyruvate (not for COMT++) and supplements entitled "Krebs cycle intermediates" (provided they do not include glutamate, aspartate or their derivatives), such as zinc in a complex with Krebs cycle intermediates. Again, testing to determine the level of various Krebs cycle intermediates should be done before deciding on which supplements to utilize.

Glutathione Support

- Glutathione Support
- CBS + or + +

When there are mutations in the GST enzyme pathway it would ordinarily make sense to supplement with sulfur donors as well as with glutathione. However where he/she has the CBS up regulation the use of sulfur donors can be a problem. Given the CBS C699T+, limiting the supplementation of glutathione to the use of the thio skin cream or another single form of glutathione that is non lipid based is the best compromise that takes into account the entire nutrigenomic profile. The CBS C699T mutation leads to the enhanced breakdown of homocysteine which generates excess sulfur groups that can be a problem for G6PDH as excessive amounts of sulfur donors can lead to decreased levels of G6PDH. If a G6PDH mutation also is present than these excess sulfur groups can aggravate the underlying issue with this enzyme.

Rather than going with the philosophy of the "more glutathione the better" it is important to temper this with an eye toward keeping glutathione supplemented but not going overboard in terms of the total number of sulfur donors in the system and keeping the CBS status in mind. Individuals with the CBS C699T+ mutation do not always tolerate lipid based supplementation well. Based on these factors you can consider the use of non lipid types of glutathione as well as a glutathione based toothpaste that may also help to address streptococcal infection in the oral cavity as well as the addition of NADH. The use of NADH should help to compensate for issues with glutathione recycling that can be caused by G6PDH deficiencies.

- Glutathione Support
- CBS - - (no upregulation)

When their are mutations in the GST enzyme pathway it would make sense to supplement with sulfur donors as well as with glutathione as this may be a factor in terms of metal accumulation in his/her system. Where he/she does not have the CBS up regulation the use of sulfur donors should not be a problem. However, excessive amounts of sulfur donors can lead to decreased levels of glucose 6 phosphate dehydrogenase (G6PDH). Rather than going with the philosophy of the "more glutathione the better" it is important to temper this with an eye toward keeping glutathione supplemented but not going overboard in terms of the total number of sulfur donors in the system and keeping G6PDH in mind. Choices for glutathione supplements would include the use of topical glutathione, oral glutathione as well as IV glutathione with the addition of NADH. The use of NADH should help to compensate for issues with glutathione recycling that can be caused by G6PDH deficiencies.

There are several different types of glutathione lozenges as well as a specially formulated GSH oral glutathione, an oral lipid based glutathione for enhanced transport and thione glutathione cream. In addition there is a glutathione toothpaste as well as glutathione shampoo that is available. You can also consider using NAC (500mg per day), vitamin C with rose hips (500mg two to three times per day), vitamin E with mixed tocopherols, and selenium. These supplements will help to maintain and regenerate healthy glutathione levels without directly adding too many sulfur groups. The HHC neurological health general vitamin includes low doses of several sulfur donors such as taurine, broccoli extract and garlic which will also be beneficial. The use of any combination of these products would be suitable for him/her.

In summary, you should consider one or two sources of glutathione on a daily basis. In addition a glutathione based toothpaste may also help to address streptococcal infection in the oral cavity.

Gut, Thyroid, Sinus, & Pancreatic Support

- Gut, Sinus, Thyroid, & Pancreatic Support

The use of vitamin C and Biotene toothpaste or mouthwash (available at your local pharmacy) may also aid the mitochondria in detoxification and help to support SOD and glutathione mutations. The Biotene toothpaste, mouthwash and gum may also be useful in combating chronic streptococcal infection. Many individuals have issues with chronic streptococcal infection or chronic issues with other bacterial infections in the body. In addition chronic gut issues can indicate an underlying bacterial infection in his body.

Streptococcal infection in the gut can serve as a reservoir to reinfect the sinuses. Chronic streptococcal infection has been associated with OCD behavior as well as tics, over stimulatory behavior and perseverative speech. Streptococcal infection can also lay the groundwork for leaky gut which can relate to decreased weight gain or slower growth.

Xylitol nasal spray will help to eliminate nasal strep, reduce ear infections and has been reported to help with leaky gut, most likely by deceasing the flow of streptococci from the sinuses into the gut. Xylitol is also available as a sugar for cooking and in Biotene gum, toothpaste and mouthwash. Another tip is to add in papaya enzyme with increased doses of vitamin C. This helps to support the body to eliminate chronic sinus issues as well as the reservoir of strep in the gut. I suggest that you use as much papaya enzyme and vitamin C as your body can tolerate without causing loose stools. ImmunFactor 5 once every other day will aid the body in addressing the bacterial issues as well as the use of Microbial Support RNA on a daily basis. The supplement IP6 may help to reduce stimulatory behaviors and OCD behaviors associated with chronic streptococcal infection as will the use of benfotiamine. The use of lactoferrin is also excellent to support the body in addressing streptococcal and other bacterial issues as it helps to limit the availability of iron for the microbes. Many microbes require the presence of iron for growth and/or virulence.

Aside from the toxic effects of mercury on the body, aluminum and lead toxicity can cause toxicity in the body. Bacteria seem to be able to hold onto aluminum. Aluminum is known to inhibit glutamate dehydrogenase which is an enzyme that converts glutamate to alpha keto glutarate. In addition aluminum interferes with the production of BH4. Therefore the presence of aluminum may be affecting levels of serotonin as well as dopamine in the body and may be affecting BH4 levels regardless of whether there is an MTHFR A1298C mutation. Malic acid, EDTA and horsetail grass are all helpful in binding aluminum in the body. As chronic bacterial infection is addressed it should help to aid in aluminum excretion.

As already mentioned the gut may be a source or reservoir for chronic bacterial infection if it is an issue in the body. There are a number of herbs that are useful in supporting the body to address bacterial imbalances in the gut .One natural mixture that appears to work includes neem, myrrh, golden seal, cranberry, Oregon grape, barberry, uva ursi; using ½ to one whole capsule of each three times per day for one month. If a CDSA test indicates that organisms are resistant to any of these natural herbs a substitution can be made such that the resistant herbs in question can be replaced in the mixture with caprylic acid or oregamax. Using a mixture of herbs such as these seven or more herbs simultaneously is less likely to lead to resistance than using single herbs to support the body in addressing microbial issues.

Cranberry is also excellent for support for the body to address E.coli and neem is supportive for parasites as well as for bacterial issues. Low levels of BH4 as a result of high aluminum in the body or as a result of mutations (MTHFR A1298C or CBSC699T) can lead to more severe parasitic infections. The use of Paradex is also helpful for supporting the body to address parasites.

It is also important to support normal flora. One successful strategy is to rotate the normal flora to get a good mixture and variety. Preferred sources of normal flora include suprema dophilus, inuflora, kyodophilus, Ultra dairy support (even if you are not eating dairy this is a good source of flora), a sprinkle of Toueff, Colon Health Support and allerdophilus and IMF #7. If possible use ½ to one whole capsule of a different source of normal flora each day of the week. You can also use the Mycology Support RNA and Candex once a day, as well as the Bowel Support and Stomach pH RNA to help to balance the gut. By following this plan, you create an environment where the normal flora can thrive and as a result you will help to eliminate the offending organisms. At the end of a month it is a wise idea to run a complete diagnostic stool analysis (CDSA) to confirm that the gut flora is in balance.

Loose stools are an issue for a number of individuals, and I do understand that the SCD (Specific Carbohydrate Diet) has made a big difference in these cases. However, if you are supplementing protein it is important to monitor ammonia levels to be certain that the body is able to dispose of the ammonia properly that are generated from the intake of high protein foods. The body uses two molecules of BH4 to detoxify one molecule of ammonia to urea. This is an expensive way to use your BH4. BH4 is also needed for dopamine and serotonin as well as language related function. Since language is a primary problem for many children, using up limited BH4 to detoxify ammonia may not be the best use of it for the body. In addition, ammonia is reported to inhibit he metabolism of butyrate, along with other short chain fatty acids. Butyrate is a nutrient used by cells that line the gut.

Butyrate synthesis can be inhibited by H2S and sulfites that are generated as a result of the CBS up regulation, low molybdenum or SUOX mutations. Paradoxically butyrate has been reported to be a potent detoxifier of ammonia.

Excess stomach acid in the system can cause loose stools and severe stomach pain. Ammonia that is generated from excessive protein is alkaline. This may help to neutralize the stomach acid and would make the stools and gut pain better. However, using a high protein diet to address loose stools is not dealing with the root of the problem if it is caused by excess stomach acid. Creating high ammonia levels via diet to neutralize acids treats the symptom but not the underlying imbalance in the body. Stomach acid is triggered by histamine reacting with H2 receptors in the stomach. So a high protein diet may be increasing ammonia which is neutralizing the stomach acid and improving the gut issue. However, it is not addressing why you have excess acid in the first place nor is it considering why there may be high histamine in the system (histamine is related to methylation function). In addition it is important to evaluate ammonia levels and to consider the consequences of high ammonia. I am not suggesting that individuals abandon the SCD diet, especially as it has made a positive difference for many people. However, I would suggest a test for Helicobacter pylori as that is often a causative agent for excess stomach acid. The use of mastica gum is reported to be very helpful for addressing this organism. I would suggest ½ mastica gum, Stomach pH and Bowel support with meals. I would also suggest that you consider running a DDI urine amino acid test so that you can look at ammonia levels and amino acids while on the SCD diet.

On a related note other helpful tools for addressing bacterial and viral infection and supporting the body in the process include the use of Ora Triplex, Immuno Forte, Moducare and the ImmunFactors (IMF). In particular IMF 4 should be helpful for viruses related to childhood vaccines. The IMF 1, 2 and 6 should be helpful in supporting the body for herpes related viruses and I have found that the IMF 5 works nicely for support for bacterial infections. Those individuals with CBS C699T+ mutations should limit their use of IMFs to one per day due to lipid acting components in the product.

In animal models vitamin B2 (riboflavin) has been shown to speed the clearance of bacteria from the body and to lower mortality rates from bacterial sepsis. In addition, riboflavin is reported to be helpful in reducing inflammatory mediators. Another B vitamin, vitamin B3, is often depleted in individuals with chronic bacterial infections. You may also want to consider niacinamide (1/2 per day) as this may help to stem the breakdown of tryptophan that is often seen with bacterial infection. Kynurenate is part of the breakdown pathway for

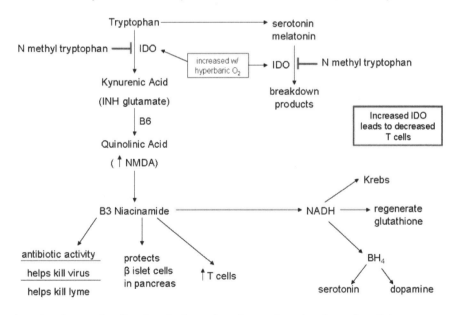

tryptophan. As the body breaks down tryptophan for this purpose it will also deplete serotonin. Lack of serotonin combined with streptococcal infection can lead to perseverative and OCD behaviors in addition to other effects. The final breakdown product of the tryptophan pathway is niacinamide. This B vitamin has been reported to have antimicrobial effects. It may be that the body is trying to address bacterial infection by breaking down tryptophan into niacinamide to help with infection.

In some cases I have not found that the use of high dose B6 or P5P is always helpful. It can actually cause more overstimulatory or OCD type behaviors. While kynurenic acid is calming for neurotransmitters, the product that kynurenines are converted to by B6 is quinolinic acid. Quinolinic acid is an excitotoxin. So if you have high kynurenine and add B6 you can generate quinolinic acid which acts as an excitotoxin and can aggravate the nervous system. Increased levels of quinolinic acid have been implicated in Alzheimer's disease as well as with respect to excitotoxin damage of nerves.

Quinolinic acid was found to be substantially elevated in patients with Borrelia burgdorferi (Lyme) infection and has been postulated to play a role in contributing to neurological and cognitive defects associated with Lyme disease.

It is of importance to try to look at why you may have elevated activity in the tryptophan breakdown pathway in the first place. Decreased methylation, increased IDO (an enzyme that is also effected by methylation and other factors), and chronic streptococcal or even B. burgdorferi (lyme) infection can lead to stimulation of this pathway.

A future consideration may be to look at addressing the possibility of chronic Lyme infection in the body. Lyme disease has been implicated in a number of neurological conditions. Cat's claw is reported to be helpful for viral issues as well as for Lyme. Artemisia (wormwood) has also shown activity against Lyme. Wormwood is a component of Paradex that was already mentioned with respect to other parasitic infections. In addition, tick support RNAs and IMF 2 should help to support the body.

Periodic thyroid tests and CDSAs to assess the status of bacterial infection and it effect on thyroid function are suggested for individuals who have issues with chronic bacterial infection, sinus infections, dental issues, or a past history of ear infections

One of the enzymes that is activated during chronic bacterial infection can also deplete tyrosine levels. The amino acid tyrosine is a precursor for both thyroid hormones as well as for dopamine synthesis. If tyrosine levels are being depleted he/she may be having dopamine issues in spite of the COMT and VDR Bsm/Taq status. While this may not be an issue, again, this is a good time to raise potential problems so that you can be aware of them and watch for signs of these on future tests. Low thyroid function can be associated with chronic sinus infections. It is a good idea to check thyroid status particularly in individuals with chronic bacterial or sinus infections as are often found in association with a variety of neurological and cardiovascular conditions. Natural thyroid supplementation is available in the form of thyroid/tyrosine supplements. Iodine levels also affect thyroid function and there is a relationship between the methylation cycle, sulfur groups and iodine levels. Iodine levels will be impacted negatively by bromine that is used in bread. This is another reason to be vigilant with the gluten free aspect of the GF/CF diet. Lithium is concentrated in the thyroid and can inhibit iodine uptake. This is why it is important to monitor both the levels of iodine as well as lithium on essential mineral tests and supplement only as needed for low values that may occur as a result of detoxification and excretion of mercury.

If thyroid hormone levels are an issue, the use of ½ to one Iodoral per day may be of help in supporting healthy iodine levels. The use of the herb guggul may help to balance T3 and T4. After four weeks of nutritional support you should run a follow up thyroid test with your health care provider to confirm that thyroid hormone levels are in the normal range and an essential mineral test to confirm healthy iodine levels (or the use of the topical iodine test). The thyroid hormone iodination cycle is tied to glucose 6 phosphate dehydrogenase levels. G6PDH levels are affected by sulfur groups. As thyroid issues are addressed it can help to clear the chronic bacterial/sinus infections in the body.

Chronic streptococcal infection, and possibly E.coli infection can lead to a variety of inflammatory mediators as well as depleting neurotransmitters. Bacterial infection is also known to increase the levels of inflammatory mediators such as IL6 and TNF alpha. Mutations have been characterized that aid in increasing the levels IL6 or TNF alpha in the system. Elevated IL6 has been reported to inhibit the release of thyroid hormones in addition to its role in enhancing inflammation. The use of Health Foundation RNA, vitamin K, Kidney Support RNA, nettle, boswellia, Behavior Support RNAs and skullcap may help to balance the body so that these mediators are less of an issue. In addition curcumin and green tea may be helpful for COMT - - individuals.

In addition to its reported effect on IL6, vitamin K may also be useful in supporting blood sugar imbalances. The Fok + + marker for the VDR (vitamin D receptor) has been associated with potential blood sugar issues. Vitamin D levels are also closely tied to a variety of neurological conditions. Based on recent literature individuals should consider supplementing with at least 1000 IU of supplemental vitamin D daily. Also the use of ¼ dropper of ProLongevity RNA has proven to be helpful for many individuals. Vitamin K and supplements to support the pancreas should also be considered such as OraPancreas, Gymnema sylvestre and Super Digestive enzymes. It would also be wise to monitor levels of chromium on an essential mineral test and consider supplementation if levels are low. In addition, to effects on blood sugar, variations in the VDR Fok marker reflect differences in bone mineral density. While increased bone mineral density is associated with increased calcium absorption it has also been associated with higher blood concentrations of lead.

In addition to effects on blood sugar levels, decreased pancreatic activity may be associated with increased levels of oxalic acid as measured on organic acid tests. Supplementation to support healthy blood sugar levels and the pancreas may also be helpful in normalizing increased oxalic acid. In addition the use of the herbs Sheep sorrel and Turkey rhubarb may contribute to elevated levels of oxalic acid.

On a related note, pantothenic acid and quercetin (not for COMT +) may be helpful for elevated uric acid along with supplementation to support the kidneys (Kidney Support RNA, OraKidney, dandelion leaf).

ACE mutations and Sodium/Potassium Levels

- Ace Support

Mutations can occur that affect the activity of the ACE (angiotensin converting enzyme). Up regulations in activity of this enzyme lead to higher than expected conversion of angiotensin I to angiotensin II. High levels of angiotensin II in turn increase the level of aldosterone. High levels of aldosterone lead to decreased excretion of sodium in the urine and increased excretion of potassium in the urine. This suggests that low sodium and high potassium on a urine essential element test may reflect aldosterone excess and may indicate ACE up regulations. In animal studies high levels of angiotensin II were correlated with increased anxiety and decreases in learning and memory.

Support for ACE mutations in this pathway can include Kidney Support RNA, OraKidney, OraAdrenal, Stress and Anxiety Support RNA. BioNativus multiminerals can be used for a general mineral support.

Aldosterone can also be regarded as a stress hormone as its levels are elevated in the blood following stressful situations. Consequently, even in the absence of an ACE upregulation, situations of chronic stress can result in increased levels of aldosterone causing sodium retention and increased potassium excretion. This excess potassium is excreted provided that the kidneys are functioning properly. In the event that kidney function is compromised, it can lead to the retention of potassium in the body.

While the initial effect of increased aldosterone is the retention of sodium and increased secretion of potassium, over time, as the adrenals become fatigued and unable to release adequate amounts of aldosterone and/or cortisol the levels of potassium start to rise and sodium levels may begin to fall in the body. When this occurs it can result in increased retention of potassium.

In cases of imbalances in sodium and potassium excretion it is worthwhile to consider adrenal and kidney support. Also reducing stress is helpful as aldosterone is basically acting like a stress hormone.

General support for the adrenals and kidneys in the absence of specific ACE mutations includes OraKidney, OraAdrenal, Stress and Kidney Support RNA.

On a related note, licorice is often used for a number of healing purposes. It should be recognized, however, that licorice inhibits enzymes that break down aldosterone and cortisol and so its use may be non ideal for those with imbalances in these regions. The use of licorice can lead to increased levels of aldosterone. Licorice can also cause an increased craving for salt, loss of potassium and increased water intake. This may be related to its inhibition of the enzyme11 beta hydroxysteroid dehydrogenase. Grapefruit juice also inhibits the activity of this enzyme.

Phosphatidyl serine is reported to help to control excess cortisol in the body in addition to its role in the back door synthesis of methionine.

Additional Resources

Specific information about supplements discussed in this book can be obtained at www.holisiticheal.com

Dr. Amy's personal website is www.holistichealth.com

Dr. Amy answers questions at www.ch3nutrigenomics.com

Video Tapes/DVDs & Books that are divided by topic:

- **Glutamate and Gaba**
    - Neurological Inflammation, *Video Tape*

- **Virus, Metals, Methylation**
    - Austin Conference, November 2004 *DVD*
    - Phoenix Conference, April 2005 *DVD*

- **Factors Contributing to Autism**
    - Putting It All Together Parents Weekend, *Video Tape or DVD*
    - Boston Conference, August 2004 *DVD*
    - The Puzzle of Autism, *Book*
    - Dr. Amy's Supplement Guide, *DVD*
    - Autism Educational Starter Package

- **RNA**
    - Boston Conference, August 2004, *DVD*
    - Phoenix Conference, April 2005, *DVD*
    - Heal Your Body Naturally, *Book*
    - RNA Educational Starter Package

Concluding Thoughts

Those of you reading this book who have interacted directly with me know that I am a very spiritual person. I think it is important to keep in mind the spiritual aspect of healing as much as the biochemical aspects of healing.

This point is illustrated by a question concerning the use of gold salts by one of the parents of an autistic child on the chat room. I first learned of the use of gold salts for autism though this parent, which helps to reinforce the idea that as doctors and researchers we do not have the market on information. I think it is always important to keep our minds open to new ideas and to remember that no matter how much we think we know there is so much more to learn. While I do not know if this therapy works I will be open to watching what the results show. On a practical side I have concerns about adding metals to a system that is already over burdened with metals. However from a spiritual standpoint I am intrigued. For a long time now I have wondered "when the gold would show up". The three wise men brought frankincense, gold and myrrh. Frankincense is the same as boswellia. Boswellia is an herb with anti inflammatory activity. Myrrh is a wonderful, natural antimicrobial and I have been wondering about when gold would have a role. So, I will be open to considering the use of gold salts for inflammation. I believe that we always need to balance the practical science with the spiritual possibilities.

Just as I began this book with an excerpt from the book Heal Your Body Naturally: The Power of RNA (Dr. Amy Yasko and Dr. Garry Gordon) I would also like to conclude this book with a excerpt. This second excerpt illustrates that even when we are talking about something so biochemically tangible as DNA and genetics, that there is much in the Universe for all of us to learn.

Excerpt from Heal Your Body Naturally: The Power of RNA
By Dr. Amy Yasko and Dr. Garry Gordon

"Dr.Craig Venter is president of one of the firms that led the Human Genome Project. He is quoted as remarking that *"We have only 300 unique genes in the human genome that are not in the mouse. This tells me genes can't possibly explain all of what makes us what we are."* This statement from an individual so intimately involved in the molecular biology and biotechnology of DNA sequences suggests that we need to look beyond the mere "spelling" of our DNA and RNA when it comes to our health.

Dr. Larry Dossey writes about three Eras of medicine that have progressed since the mid 19th century. Dr. Yasko simply describes "Era I "medicine as "if this, then that" medicine. This would include taking a specific herb to remedy a specific condition or an antibiotic to eradicate a bacterial infection.

According to Dr. Dossey *"Era I is good old everyday mechanical medicine, technical orthodox medicine. Drugs, surgery and radiation. Era I, which can be called "mechanical medicine" and which began roughly in the 1860s, reflects the prevailing view that health and illness are totally physical in nature, and thus all therapies should be physical ones, such as surgical procedures or drugs* "(Dossey, L, Reinventing Medicine, HarperCollins Publishers, 1999).

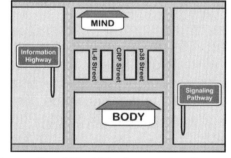

Era II medicine is how your mind affects your body. It acknowledges that stress and your frame of mind can have a negative impact on your body. It is what is commonly referred to as the Mind/Body connection.

Very specific inflammatory mediators have been well characterized in terms of their ability to convey stress to the body. Mediators such as il6, p38 Map kinase and CRP are some of the information pathways that the mind uses to convert stress into harmful effects on the body. Scientific studies have reported that higher CRP levels were found in men in their 70's with less social interaction as compared with men with more social interaction. (Bottom Line Health, June 2004). Elevated CRP is associated with levels of inflammation and is a risk factor for a number of inflammatory disorders including heart disease, colon cancer and Alzheimer's disease among others. A study published in the very prestigious journal Proceedings of the National Academy of Science in July 2003 reported that after following individuals over a six year time period, increases in IL6 have been correlated with stress. A series of papers in this same journal in July of 2004, underscored the relationship between stress and yet another inflammatory mediator, p38MAP kinase. These types of relationships between well defined concrete, measurable inflammatory mediators and the ability of the mind to trigger the release of these mediators falls under the domain of Era II medicine. Keeping that "in mind" you should never underestimate the power of spirituality or positive thoughts and the impact it can have on your health.

Patients with osteoarthritis who believed in their ability to perform tasks were less debilitated after 3 years than those who were less confident (Loucks, Bottom Line Health vol 18 June 2004). Conversely, research from McGill University (Spirituality and Health March/April 2004) has shown that brains from senior citizens with low self-esteem had atrophied leading to a higher incidence of memory loss than those who felt good about themselves. People scoring higher on anxiety tests were 25% more likely to have premalignancies (Clinical Pearls May 2004). Two separate studies support a correlation between prayer and the ability to become pregnant (Cuvelier,

M. Psychology Today, Jan. 2002). Your frame of mind, as evidenced by your spirituality, appears to increase life span (Bottom Line Health May 2004).

This mind/body effect can be very powerful even when it comes to surgery. In a study involving 30 patients, only 12 received the <u>actual</u> surgical treatment; the other 18 only received a sham surgical procedure. Neither the participants, nor the medical attending staff knew which procedure each participant received. One year later, the 10 patients who <u>thought</u> they received the transplant reported better physical, emotional, and social functioning than the 20 who <u>believed</u> they had received the sham surgery. The medical staff also reported improved outcomes in the patients who <u>believed</u> they had received the treatment. Of the 10 who were doing better, and believed they had received the actual surgical procedure, only 4 of them had in fact received the treatment. This study helps to confirm that believing in a treatment and the power of positive thinking help to make it more effective (McRae, C., Arch Gen Psychiatry. April 2004).

"Era II began to take shape in the period following World War II. Physicians began to realize, based on scientific evidence, that disease has a "psychosomatic" aspect: that emotions and feelings can influence the body's functions. Psychological stress, for example, can contribute to high blood pressure, heart attacks, and ulcers. This was a radical advance over Era I. Era II is involved any time we talk about mind/body events within the person. My mind affecting my brain affecting my body, for good or ill. It's confined to the present moment, it's "here and now "medicine, it's local." (Dossey, L. Reinventing Medicine)

Era III medicine is how "my" mind affects "your" body. This is an area that is not completely understood; yet the power of belief or prayer and its affect on healing has been proven to occur.

"*Era III is mind/body medicine with a different slant. The recently developing Era III goes even further by proposing that consciousness is not confined to one's individual body. Nonlocal mind -- mind that is boundless and unlimited - is the hallmark of Era III. An individual's mind may affect not just his or her body, but the body of another person at a distance, even when that distant individual is unaware of the effort. You can think of Era II as illustrating the personal effects of consciousness and Era III as illustrating the transpersonal effects of the mind. It's important to remember that these eras are not mutually exclusive; rather they coexist, overlap, and are used together, as when drugs are used with psychotherapy, and surgery is used with prayer.*" (Dossey, L. Reinventing Medicine)

We do know from studies being conducted around the world that there are hard facts and statistics that support the idea that Era III medicine is a reality. Studies at the Princeton Engineering Anomalies Research Laboratory have been conducted for over a decade by the ex-Dean of Engineering Dr. Robert Jahn and his colleague Brenda Dunne. In their remote-sensing experiments, the scientists had one person in Princeton attempting to mentally send a computer-selected image to a person 6000 miles away. Significantly, the receiver was able to get the message in great detail. This is mind operating outside of our conventional views of space and time.

Similar instances of distance communication are seen in nature. "*When a queen ant is spatially separated from her colony, building still continues fervently and according to plan. If the queen is killed, however, all work in the colony stops. No ant knows what to do. Apparently the queen sends the building plans*" also from far away via the group consciousness of her subjects. She can be as far away as she *wants, as long as she is alive. In man hyper communication is most often encountered when one suddenly gains access to information that is outside one's knowledge base."*

So too we know that distant prayer, or if you prefer positive thoughts or affirmations, have been shown to affect a number of health conditions. Research at Duke University Medical Center in Durham, North Carolina studied the effects of prayer on patients undergoing cardiac procedures such as catheterization and angioplasty. Patients receiving prayer had up to 100% fewer side effects from these procedures than people not prayed for (Archives of Internal Med. Oct., 1999, Krucoff, American Heart Journal, 142, 2001, Grunberg, Cardiology Rev., 2003). A recent article from the ordinarily "very Era I medical journal", the Journal of the American Medical Association, noted that seeing a loved one in pain activates some of the same brain areas that are mobilized when we experience pain ourselves (Journal American Medical Association March 17, 2004). A case of _my_ mind reacting to _your_ body.

One would need a guide to navigate uncharted areas through the African rain forest as it would be impossible to get to your destination without that guide who is familiar with the territory. Similarly, just because _we_ don't know the way to get there, does not mean that a place does not exist. In terms of Era III medicine we do not have to know exactly which roads to transverse to arrive at the final destination, just simply to acknowledge that the destination and the roads do exist. For some it is a place they would prefer not to even attempt to travel to, and we must respect that choice.

So what you might ask does all this have to do with RNA? The point is that seemingly unconventional pathways do exist even if we do not yet know what they are or we do not fully understand them. It is sufficient to be open minded and be aware that they may in fact have an impact on our health.

For those who are skeptics it should be intriguing to now learn that only 2% to 5% of the genome encodes protein. In other words as far as we know at this time only 5% of the DNA in each of our cells, that same DNA that is long enough to stretch all the way to the sun and back again, is used for anything that we would consider useful. Among the 5% that is actually used there is a high degree of similarity between diverse species. An in depth analysis of the conservation of genes between species suggests *"...the existence of a selective force in the overall design of genetic pathways to maintain a highly connected class of genes"* (Stuart, J. Science, Oct. 2003).

As described in the article "So Much Junk DNA In Our Genome" (Ono, S. Brookhaven Symp Biol. 1972) approximately 95% of our DNA is not utilized to make proteins and hence must be "junk". However, recent work has shown that this so called "junk" DNA is <u>more highly conserved</u> between species than the other 5% that is used to make proteins. The high degree of conservation between species of this other 95% suggests that there is an important function to these regions that has not yet been determined. (Dermitzakis, E. et al Science November 2003).

Former senior computer systems designer, now turned author, Gregg Braden demonstrates in his book The God Code, that *"When correlated with an ancient alphabet, the code of all life becomes a translatable message in our cells"* (Braden, G., The God Code Hay House Publishers 2004).

The role that our DNA may play in communication is confirmed by recent discoveries involving dolphins. *"Beyond being life's blueprint, DNA plays a powerful role in newly discovered communications between dolphins and humans, according to a team of Cetacean (dolphin and whale) researchers at the Sirius Institute on the Big Island of Hawaii. An ongoing study there shows these marine mammals receive and transmit sound signals capable of affecting the genetic double helix...using natural biotechnology DNA is activated, new research shows, by waves and particles of energized sound and light which, more than chemicals or drugs, switch genes "on" or "off."* (Tetrahedron, Oct. 6, 2004).

Russian scientists have taken this premise a step further. Scientists in the fields of biophysics and molecular biology have collaborated with linguists and geneticists to study this 95% "junk DNA". The results of their work suggest that DNA is not only responsible for the physical construction of the body but that it also serves as one huge data storage and communication system. The Russian linguists found that this highly conserved 95% of DNA that was apparently useless followed the same rules as all human language.

"To this end they compared the rules of syntax (the way in which words are put together to form phrases and sentences), semantics (the study of meaning in language forms) and the basic rules of grammar. They found that the alkalines of our DNA follow a regular grammar and do have set rules just like our languages " (Fosar, .G. and Bludorf, F. Vernetztw Intelligenz March 2001). The results of this work may help to explain aspects of Era III medicine as well as certain facets of clairvoyance, intuition, spontaneous and remote acts of healing.

This 95% to 98% "junk DNA" that is not utilized to make protein is a situation that may be unique to certain species. Bacteria, for instance, use the majority of their DNA for protein production. This has lead to the suggestion that the function of the majority of the DNA is to make RNAs that may be involved in communication and cellular regulation. *"Less than 2% of the*

3.2 billion bases in the human genome code for proteins...Does this suggest that the reason for the 'superiority' of humans lies in the 98% of the genome that does not code for proteins? Is it not conceivable that the end products of many mammalian genes are not proteins, but RNAs?...Is it conceivable that certain RNA molecules are the actual creators and controllers of life?" (Pieztch, J. Understanding the RNAissance, May 2003).

And so we have come full circle. Whether we quote Dr. Gary Zweiger, geneticist from Stanford and Columbia Universities, Genentech, Incyte and Agilent Technologies, "*Genes are the most obvious conveyors of information with living beings... As information it does not really matter how the gene is encoded, so long as the message can be received and decoded... Molecular messages may move a bit slower than the speed of light, but as information they are essentially no different than messages sent over phone lines or reflected off of satellites: they all may be transduced, digitized and stored.*" Or we may quote the Russian scientists "*DNA...also serves as data storage and in communication. Living chromosomes function ... like computers....*" Regardless of whom we quote we come to the same conclusion. We can take advantage of this inherent communication capability within our genes to talk to our cells for optimal health and wellness."

With love and hope and belief in good health always,
Dr. Amy

"*The inclination to goodness is imprinted deeply in the nature of man. It is our uniqueness as a species, coupled with our fundamental character of goodness that opens the door for the message in our cells to see real and lasting change in our lives.*"
(Braden, G. The God Code Hay House Publishers 2004)

About the Author

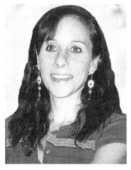

Amy A. Yasko Ph.D., ND, NHD, AMD, HHP, FAAIM, has extensive expertise in biochemistry, molecular biology, and biotechnology. She also has research and clinical experience in both allopathic and alternative medicine. The common thread that winds through these fields is her work with RNA.

As co-founder and owner of a successful biotechnology company, she is recognized as an expert in molecular biology in the field of DNA/RNA based diagnostics and therapeutics and has been a consultant to the medical and research community for eighteen years. More than twenty years ago she began isolating single copy RNA messages from transformed cells at Strong Memorial Hospital Cancer Center. Later while at Yale Medical Center she worked to enhance the expression of specific eukaryotic RNAs from yeast.

During her tenure at St. Vincent's Hospital in NYC, Dr. Yasko developed custom diets and used nutritional supplements to improve the cure rates of Hodgkin's disease patients. She worked with Dr. Lawrence to isolate some of the first clinical samples of Transfer Factor for use in these patients. She then went on to conduct molecular research on Transfer Factor in Dr. Fudenburg's Immunology Dept. at the Medical University of South Carolina.

Dr. Yasko was also a member of the Dept. of Pediatrics and Infectious Diseases at Strong Memorial Hospital and worked to develop safer *Haemophilus influenza* vaccines. She has also spent years studying the relationship between energy transport and modes of antibiotic resistance by bacteria and has written articles and chapters in books on the subject.

Dr. Yasko then established an alternative healthcare practice specializing in chronic inflammation, immunological and neurological disorders. To date she has had considerable success in halting and in most cases reversing the effects of such debilitating diseases from which her clients suffer, such as ALS, MS, Parkinson's disease, Alzheimer's disease, SLE, Myasthenia gravis and autism. Most recently her primary focus has been to construct a program to help to reverse autism.

Dr. Yasko graduated cum laude with a BS in Chemistry and Fine Arts from Colgate University. She then completed her medical education at Albany Medical College and received a Doctorate in Microbiology, Immunology and Infectious Diseases with an award for outstanding academic excellence, graduating summa cum laude. She was the first woman in that department to receive a Doctorate in this field. Dr. Yasko continued her education to graduate with high honors from the Clayton College of Natural Health, receiving two additional degrees, a Doctor of Naturopathy and a Doctor of Natural Health. She is licensed as a Naturopathic Physician and board certified as an Alternative Medical Doctor, a Holistic Health Practitioner and is a Fellow of the American Association of Integrative Medicine. She was the recipient of the 2004 CASD award for RNA Research in autism.

Dr. Yasko has coauthored two previous books, The Puzzle of Autism and Heal Your Body Naturally: The Power of RNA. She lives in Maine with her husband and three children.

References

A Simplified Description of DNA Methylation. http://dnamethysoc.server101.com.

Abernathy, Charles O. et al. Arsenic: Health Effects, Mechanisms of Actions, and Research Issues. Environmental Health Perspectives. July 1999; 107(7).

Allelic Variants. http://srs.sanger.ac.uk/srsbin/cgi-bin/wgetz

Alternation of DNA Methylation Could Be the Way to Cell Aging. www.innovitaresearch.org. June 25, 2003.

Altindag, ZZ et al. Effects of the metals on dihydropteridine reductase activity. Toxicology In Vitro. October-December 2003; 17(5-6):533-7.

Altmann P et al. Serum aluminum levels and erythrocyte dihydropteridine reductase activity in patients on hemodialysis. New England Journal of Medicine. July 9, 1987; 317(2):80-4.

Aras, O et al. Influence of 699C-->T and 1080C--> polymorphisms of the cystathionine B-synthase gene on plasma homocysteine levels. Clinical Genetics, December 2000; 53(6):455.

Arsenate Reduction and Arsenite Methylation. Arsenic in Drinking Water. Commission on Life Sciences. The National Academies Press. 1999.

Barak, AJ et al. Betaine effects on hepatic methionine metabolism elicited by short-term ethanol feeding. Alcohol. Sept-Oct. 1996; 13(5):483-6.

Bensemain, F et al. Association study of the Ornithine Transcarbamylase Gene with Alzheimer's disease. 7e Colloque de la Societe des neurosciences. Lille 2005, C.14.

Bergman, Yehudit et al. A Stepwise Epigenetic Process Controls Immunoglobulin Allelic Exclusion. Nature Reviews Immunology. October 2004; 4:753-761.

Beyer, Katrin et al. Cystathionine Beta Synthase Could Be A Risk Factor for Alzheimer Disease. Current Alzheimer Research. May 2004; 1(2):127-133.

Beyer, K et al. Methionine synthase polymorphism is a risk factor for Alzheimer disease. Neuroreport. July 18, 2003; 14(10):1391-4.

Bhave, MR et al. Methylation status and organization of the metallothionein-I gene in livers and testes of strains of mice resistant and susceptible to cadmium. Toxicology. Aug 1988; 50(3):231-45.

Bodamer OA et al. Creatine metabolism in combined methylmalonic aciduria and homocystinuria. Ann Neurology. March 22, 2005; 57(4):557-560.

Boodman, Sandra. Experts Question Rise in Pediatric Diagnosis of Bipolar Illness, a Serious Mood Disorder. Washington Post. February 15, 2005.

Bosco, P et al. Methionine synthase (MTR) 2756 (A --> G) polymorphism, double heterozygosity methionine synthase 2756 AG/methionine synthase reductase (MTRR) 66 AG, and elevated homocysteinemia are three risk factors for having a child with Down syndrome. American Journal of Medical Genetics. Sept 1, 2003; 121(3):219-24.

Bradley TJ et al. MS.Binding of aluminium ions by Staphylococcus aureus 893. Experientia. November 15, 1968; 24(11):1175-6.

Bussell, Katrin. RITs (RNA-induced initiation of transcriptional gene silencing) binding to heterochromatic loci enables RNAi machinery to function in is to destroy aberrant RNAs and generate siRNAs for heterochromatic maintenance. Nature Reviews Molecular Cell Biology. Nature Genetology. 2004; 36:1174-1180.

Chase, Daniel L. et al. Mechanism of extrasynaptic dopamine signaling in Caenorhabditis elegans. Nature Neuroscience. 2004; 7:1096-1103.

Chen, X et al. Production of the neuromodulator H2S by cystathionine beta-synthase via the condensation of cysteine and homocysteine. Journal of Biological Chemistry. Dec 10, 2004; 279(50):52082-6.

Chuikov, Sergel et al. Regulation of p53 activity through lysine methylation. Nature. November 18, 2004; 432:353-360.

Compere, SJ et al. DNA methylation controls the inducibility of the mouse metallothionein-I gene lymphoid cells. Cell. July 25, 1981; (1):233-40.

Cooney, Craig. Methylation, Epigenetics and Longevity. Life Extension Magazine, December 1998.

Costa, M. Model for the epigenetic mechanism of action of nongenotoxic carcinogens. The American Journal of Clinical Nutrition. 1995; 61:666S-669S.

Costa, Max. Molecular Mechanisms of Nickel Carcinogenesis. Biological Chemistry. 383(6), 961-967.

Cowen, Rob. Twins' gene regulation isn't identical. Science News. July 9, 2005; 168:19-20.

Crang, AJ et al. The relationship of myelin basic protein (arginine) methyltransferase to myelination in mouse spinal cord. Journal of Neurochemistry. July 1982; 39(1):244-7.

Cresenzi, Carry L. et al. Cysteine Is the Metabolic Signal Responsible for Dietary Regulation of Hepatic Cysteine Dioxygenase and Glutamate Cysteine Ligase in Intact Rats. Journal of Nutrition. September 2003; 133:2697-2702.

Cutler, P et al. The effect of lead and aluminium on rat dihydropteridine reductase. Arch. Toxicology Supplement. 1987; 11:227-30.

DNA Methylation. New England Journal of Medicine. November 20, 2003.

Dagani, Ron. Staph Favors Heme. Given a choice, pathogen prefers to get its iron from iron porphyrin in blood. Chemical and Engineering News, September 13, 2004; 7.

Davis, Cindy D et al. DNA Methylation, Cancer Susceptibility, and Nutrient Interactions. Experimental Biology and Medicine, 2004; 229:988-995.

Delgado, JM et al. Effects of arsenite on central monoamines and plasmatic levels of adrenocorticotropic hormone (ACTH) in mice. Toxicology Lett. Sept. 30, 2000; 117(1-2):61-7.

Doeker, B. M. et al. Liquorice, growth retardation and Addison's disease. Horm. Res. 1999; 52(5):253-5.

Du Vigneaud, Vincent et al. The Utilization of the Methyl Group of Methionine in the Biological Synthesis of Choline and Creatine. Journal of Biological Chemistry. August 1, 1941; 140:625-641.

Dunn, Barbara K. One Side of a Larger Picture. Annals of New York Academy of Sciences, 2003; 983:28-42.

Epigenetic Effects on Individual Susceptibility to Heavy Metal- and Polycyclic Aromatic Hydrocarbon-induced DNA Damage. National Cancer Institute, Division of Cancer Prevention.

Epigenetics in Cancer Prevention: Early Detection and Risk Assessment. National Cancer Institute, Division of Cancer Prevention. Annals of New York Academy of Sciences. 2003; 983:1-4.

Erbe, Richard W et al. Severe Methylenetetrahydrofolate Reductase Deficiency, Methionine Synthase, and Nitrous Oxide—A Cautionary Tale. New England Journal of Medicine. July 3, 2003; 349(1):4-6.

Eto, K et al. A novel enhancing mechanism for hydrogen sulfide-producing activity of cystathionine beta-synthase. Journal of Biological Chemistry. Nov. 8, 2002; 277(45):42680-5.

Eussen, Simone J. P. M. et al. Oral Cyanocobalamin Supplementation in Older People with Vitamin B12 Deficiency. May 23, 2005; 265(10).

Ferguson-Smith, A.C. et al. DNA methylation in genomic imprinting, development, and disease. The Journal of Pathology. September 2001; 195(1):97-110.

Flo, TH et al. Lipocalin 2 mediates an innate immune response to bacterial infection by sequestrating iron. Nature. December 16, 2004; 7019:917-21.

Freed, WJ et al. Prevention of strychnine-induced seizures and death by the N-methylated glycine derivatives betaine, dimethylglycine sarcosine. Pharmacological Biochemistry and Behavior, April 1985; 22(4):641-3.

Freitag, Michael et al. DNA Methylation Is Independent of RNA Interference in Neurospora. Science. June 2004; 304:1939.

Funseth, E et al. Effects of coxsackievirus B3 infection on the acute-phase protein metallothionein and on cytochrome P-4501A1 involved in the detoxification processes of TCDD in the mouse. Sci. Total Environ. February 4, 2002; 284(1-3):37-47.

Funseth, E et al. Relation between trace element levels in plasma and myocardium during coxsackievirus B3 myocarditis in the mouse. Biometals. December 2000; 13(4):361-7.

Funseth, E et al. Trace element changes in the myocardium during coxsackievirus B3 myocarditis in the mouse. Biol Trace Elem Res. August 2000; 76(2):149-60.

Geiss, Gk et al. Global impact of influenza virus on cellular pathways is mediated by both replication-dependent and -independent events. Journal of Virology. May 2001; 75(9):4321-31.

Glynn, AW et al. The intestinal absorption of cadmium increases during a common viral infection (coxsackie virus B3) in mice. Chem Biol Interact. May 1, 1998; 113(1):79-89.

Gorbunova, Vera et al. Genome-Wide Demethylation Destabilizes CTG.CAG Trinucleotide Repeats in Mammalian Cells. HMG Advance Access, Sept. 30, 2004.

Ghoshal, K et al. Influenza virus infection induces metallothionein gene expression in the mouse liver and lung by overlapping but distinct molecular mechanisms. Molecular Cell Biology. December 2001; 21(24):8301-17.

Gramsbergen, Jan Bert et al. Glutathione depletion in nigrostriatal slice cultures: GABA loss, dopamine resistance and protection by the tetrahydrobiopterin precursor sepiapterin. Brain Research. May 10, 2002; 935:47-58.

Greaves, Kim et al. Prevalence of Myocarditis and Skeletal Muscle Injury During Acute Viral Infection in Adults. Archives of Internal Medicine. January 27, 2003; 263(2):165-68.

Halperin J. J. et al. Neuroactive kynurenines in Lyme borreliosis. Neurology. January 1992; 42(1):43-50.

Harding, Cary O. et al. The fate of intravenously administered tetrahydrobiopterin and its implications for heterologous gene therapy of phenylketonuria. Molecular Genetics and Metabolism. 2004; 81:52-57.

Haynes, Erin N. et al. Vitamin D Receptor Fok1 Polymorphism and Blood Lead Concentration in Children. Environmental Health Perspectives, October 2003; III(13).

Ilback, NG et al. A common viral infection can change nickel target organ distribution. Toxicology Applied Pharmacology. May 1992;114(1):166-70.

Ilback, NG et al. Altered distribution of 109cadmium in mice during viral infection. Toxicology. 1992; 71(3):193-202.

Ilback, NG. Altered distribution of heavy metals and lipids in coxsackievirus B3 infected mice. Scand J Infect Dis Suppl. 1993; 88:93-8.

Ilback, NG et al. Effects of methyl mercury on cytokines, inflammation and virus clearance in a common infection (coxsackie B3 myocarditis). Toxicol Lett. December 1996; 89(1):19-28.

Ilback, NG et al. Effects of selenium supplementation on virus-induced inflammatory heart disease. Biol Trace Elem Res. July 1998; 63(1):51-66.

Ilback, NG et al. Immune responses and resistance to viral-induced myocarditis in mice exposed to cadmium. Chemosphere. September 1994; 29(6):1145-54.

Ilback, NG et al. New aspects of murine coxsackie B3 myocarditis--focus on heavy metals. Eur Heart J. December 1995;16 (Suppl) O:20-4.

Ilback, NG et al. Metallothionein is induced and trace element balance changed in target organs of a common viral infection. Toxicology. July 1, 2004; 199(2-3):241-50.

Ilback, NG et al. Sequential changes in Fe, Cu, and Zn in target organs during early Coxsackievirus B3 infection in mice. Biol Trace Elem Res. February 9, 2003; 91(2):111-24.

Ilback, NG et al. Trace element changes in the pancreas during viral infection in mice. Pancreas. March 2003; 26(2):190-6.

Ilback, NG et al. Trace element distribution in heart tissue sections studied by nuclear microscopy is changed in Coxsackie virus B3 myocarditis in methyl mercury-exposed mice. Biol Trace Elem Res. Winter 2000; 78(1-3):131-47.

Kim, S et al. Studies on myelin basic protein-specific protein methylase I in various dysmyelinating mutant mice. Biochemical and Biophysical Research Communications. September 17, 1984. 123(2):468-74.

Krieg, Arthur M. A role for Toll in autoimmunity. Nature Immunology. 2002; 3:423-424

Kruger, Warren et al. Analysis of Functional Variation in Human Metabolic Genes. http://www.fccc.edu/research/reports/current/kruger.html. 2001.

Jiang, YH et al. A Mixed Epigenetic/Genetic Model for Oligogenic Inheritance of Autism with a Limited Role for UBE3A. American Journal of Medical Genetics, September 2004; 131A(1):1-10.

Jorgensen, Erik M. Dopamine: should I stay or should I go now? Nature Neuroscience 7. 2004; 1019-1021.

Junnila, M. et al. Betaine reduces hepatic lipidosis induced by carbon tetrachloride in Sprague-Dawley Rats. Vet Hum Toxicology. Oct 1998; 40(5):263-6.

Kauwell, Gail P. A. Emerging Concepts in Nutrigenomics: A Preveiw of What Is To Come. Nutrition in Clinical Practice. 2005;20(1):75-87.

Lamers, Yvonne et al. Supplementation with [6S]-5-methyltetrahydrofolate or folic acid equally reduces plasma total homocysteine concentrations in healthy women. American Journal of Clinical Nutrition. 2004; 79:473-478.

Langman, LJ et al. The prevalence and linkage disequilibrium of three methylenetetrahydrofolate reductase (MTHFR) gene polymorphisms varies in different ethnic groups. INABIS '98.

Lao, Jose I. et al. The Homocysteine Pathway: A New Target for Alzheimer Disease Treatment? Drug Development Research. 2004; 62(3):221-230.

Lazarus, JH. The effects of lithium therapy on thyroid and thyrotropin-releasing hormone. Thyroid. October 1998; 8(10):909-13.

Lee, Kim S. et al Deprenyl, a therapeutic agent for Parkinson's disease, inhibits arsenic toxicity protentiated by gsh depletion via inhibition of jnk activation. Journal of Toxicology Environmental Health A. 2004; 67(23-24):2013-24.

Lee, YW et al. Effects of nickel on DNA methyltransferase activity and genomic DNA methylation levels. Mutation research/Genetic Toxicology & Environmental Mutagenesis. July 31, 1998; 415(3):213-18.

Lertratanangkoon K et al. Methyl-donor deficiency due to chemically induced glutathione depletion. Cancer Research, 1996; 56(5):995-1005.

Li, K et al. Cellular response to conditional expression of hepatitis C virus core protein in Huh7 cultured human hepatoma cells. Hepatology. May 2002; 35(5):1237-46.

Li, S et al. Environmental exposure, DNA methylation, and gene regulation: lessons from diethylstilbesterol-induced cancers. Annals of New York Academy of Sciences. March 2003; 983:161-9.

Lin TS et al. Synthesis and biological activities of chloroethylurea, methylurea, and nitrosourea analogues of N-deacetylmethylthiocolchicine. Journal of Medical Chemistry. December 23, 1980; 23(12):1440-2.

Little, J et al. Colorectal neoplasia and genetic polymorphisms associated with folate metabolism. European Journal of Cancer Prevention. February 2002; 11(1):105-110.

Liver Detoxification. www.tuberose.com.

Majeed, Kazi Imran. Hyperammonemia. www.emedicine.com/neuro/topic12.htm.

McCabe, Dale C. et al. DNA Methylation, Genomic Silencing, and Links to Nutrition and Cancer. Nutrition Reviews. June 2005; 63(1):183-195, 6.

McKay, J.A. Folate and DNA Methylation During In Utero Development and Aging. Biochemical Society Transactions, 2004; 32(6):1006-7.

McLaren, D. S. Malnutrition and eye disease in Tanganyika. Nutrition and the Eye. 1960; 19(1):89-91.

Miller, L. L., Phd. et al. Liver Injury, Liver Protection, and Sulfur Metabolism: Methionine Protects Against Chloroform Liver Injury Even When Given After Anesthesia. The Journal of Experimental Medicine. 1942; 76:421-435.

Minski, Bonnie C. The Future of Nutrition is Here. Health Conscious. July 2004.

Mitchell, Brett et al. Glucocorticoid-Induced Hypertension and Tetrahydrobiopterin (BH4), a Common Cofactor for the Production of Vasoactive Molecules. Current Hypertension Reviews. January 2005; 1(1):1-6.

Nakamuro, Katsuhiko et al. Metabolism of Selenamino Acids and Contribution of Selenium Methylation to Their Toxicity. Journal of Health Science. 2002; 46(6):418-421.

Nakamuro, Katsuhiko et al. Preferential resistance of dopaminergic neurons to glutathione depletion in a reconstituted nigrostriatal system. Brain Research. 2000; 873: 203-211.

Nakamuro, Katsuhiko et al. Preferential resistance of dopaminergic neurons to the toxicity of glutathione depletion is independent of cellular glutathione peroxidase and is mediated by tetrahydrobiopterin. Journal of Neurochemistry. June 2000; 74(6):2305-14.

O'Leary, VB et al. Analysis of methionine synthase reductase polymorphisms for neural tube defects risk association. Molecular Genetic Metab. July 2005; 85(3):220-7.

Palermo, M et al. Grapefruit juice inhibits 11 beta-hydroxysteroid dehydrogenase in vivo, in mar. Clinical Endocrinology. 2003; 59(2):143-4.

Paulsen M.[1] et al. DNA methylation in genomic imprinting, development, and disease. The Journal of Pathology. September 2001; 195(1):97-110(14).

Pritzker, LB et al. Deimination of myelin basic protein. 2. Effect of methylation of MBP on its deimination by peptidylarginine deiminase. Biochemistry. May 9, 2000; 39(18):5382-8.
Pryke, LC et al. Branched chain amino acid supplementation for urea cycle disorders. www.geneswest-hgsa2004.org.

Puchacz, E et al. Vitamin D and Dopamine. Molecular Brain Research. February 1996; 36(1):193-6.

Qadura, Mohammad. Interaction of Mercury with DNA Methyltransferase. Honour's Thesis. 2004.

Razin, A. CpG methylation, chromatin structure and gene silencing-a three-way connection. EMBO J. September 1, 1998; 17(17):4905-8.

Richardson, Bruce. Biography. www.med.umich.edu/geriatrics.

Richardson, Bruce C. Role of DNA Methylation in the Regulation of Cell Function: Autoimmunity, Aging and Cancer. Journal of Nutrition. 2002; 132:2401S-2405S.

Robertson, Keith. DNA Methylation and Human Disease. Nature Reviews Genetics. August 2005; 6:597.

Santamaria-Araujo, Jose Angel et al. The Tetrahydropyranopterin Structure of the Sulfur-free and Metal-free Molybdenum Cofactor Precursor. The Journal of Biological Chemistry. April 16, 2004; 279:15994-15999.

Sarg, Bettina et al. Histone H4 Hyperacetylation Precludes Histone H4 Lysine 20 Trimethylation. Journal of Biological Chemistry. September 28, 2004; Vol. 279(51):53458-53464.

Secko, D.M. et al. The Cell Cycle: A Universal Cellular Division Program. http://www.bioteach.ubc.ca.

Siciliano, S. D. et al. Methyltransferase: an enzyme assay for microbial methylmercury formation in acidic soils and sediments. Environ Toxicol Chem. 21(6):1184-90.

Sivendran, S. et al. Two novel mutant human adenylosuccinate lyases associated with autism and characterization of the equivalent mutant B. subtilis ASL. Journal of Biological Chemistry. 2004; 10:1074.

Skinner, Michael K. Transgenerational effects of environmental toxins require an epigenetic alteration of the germ-line. Study Summary. Science. June 3, 2005; 308(5727):1466-1469.

South PK et al. Mortality in mice infected with an amyocarditic coxsackievirus and given a subacute dose of mercuric chloride.

Journal of Toxicol. Environ. Health A. August 10, 2001; 63(7):511-23.

Stipanuk, MH et al. Cysteine is the metabolic signal responsible for dietary regulation of cysteine dioxygenase and glutamate cysteine ligase in vivo. Journal of Nutrition. 2003; 133:2697-2702.

Stipanuk, MH et al. Regulation of cysteine dioxygenase and y-glutamylcysteine synthetase is associated with hepatic cysteine level. Journal of Nutritional Biochemistry. 2004; 15:112-122.

Stampfer Ma J. et al. Methylenetetrahydrofolate reductase polymorphism, dietary interactions, and risk of colorectal cancer. Cancer Research. March 15, 1997; 57(6):1098-102.

Starr, J. M. et al. Vitamin B-12, serum folate, and cognitive change between 11 and 79 years. Journal of Neurology Neurosurgery and Psychiatry. 2005; 76:291-292.

Stone, T. W. et al. The role of kynurenines in the production of neuronal death, and the neuroprotective effect of purines. Journal of Alzheimer's Disease. 2001;3(4):355-366.

Temmerman S et al. Methylation-dependent T cell immunity to Mycobacterium tuberculosis heparin-binding hemagglutinin. Nature Medicine. September 2004; 10(9):935-41. Epub August 8, 2004.

Toyosawa, T. et al. Highly purified vitamin B2 presents a promising therapeutic strategy for sepsis and septic shock. Infection and Immunity. 2004; 72:1820-1823.

Trimethylglycine TMG Overview. Life Extension. www.lef.org

Ulrey, Clayton, L. et al. The impact of metabolism on DNA methylation. Human Molecular Genetics. 2005; 14 (suppl):R139-R147.

Ulrich C. M. et al. Pharmacogenetics and folate metabolism—a promising direction. Pharmogenetics. May 2002; 3(3):299-313(15).

Uthus, Eric et al. Dietary Arsenic Affects Dimethylhydrazine Aberrant Crypt Formation and Hepatic Global DNA Methylation and Global DNA Methyltransferase Activity in Rats. USDA Agricultural Research Service. February 1, 2005.

Volpe, Arturo M. et al. Anxiety and Depression. http://www.doctorvolpe.com/anxiety.html.

Wang Jing et al. A local mechanism mediates NAD-dependent protection of axon degeneration. The Journal of Cell Biology, online July 2005.

Waterland, Robert A. et al. Transposable Elements: Targets for Early Nutritional Effects on Epigenetic Gene Regulation. Molecular and Cellular Biology, August 2003; 23(15):5293-5300.

Weaver, I. C. G. et al. Epigenetic programming by maternal behavior. Nature Neuroscience. June 2004; 27.

Weitzman, Jonathan. Targeted Methylation--Introducing methylated DNA at specific genomic loci affects local histone acetylation. Genome. Biology.com. Dec. 21, 2000.

Yung, R et al. Unexpected effects of heterozygous dnmtl null mutation on age-dependent DNA hypomethylation and autoimmunity. Journal of Gerontology. June 2001; 56(6):B268-76.

Zakharyan, RA et al. Arsenite methylation by methylvitamin B12 and glutathione
does not require an enzyme. Toxicology Applied Pharmacology. February 1, 1999; 154(3):287-91.